LAUREL ROBERTS

Quick Home Workouts for Women with Bad Knees

15-Minute Knee-Friendly Workouts for Stability, Weight Loss, Strength and Energy

Contents

1

Introduction

Hello and welcome! If you're reading this, chances are we have something in common—we've both faced the challenge of knee pain. I'm not a doctor, a personal trainer, or a TV personality. I'm just like you, a middle-aged woman navigating the complexities of life with the added hurdle of knee discomfort.

In 2019, I embarked on the journey to become a homeowner in Austin, Texas. With knee pain as my unwelcome companion, I decided on a new build and hopped from neighborhood to neighborhood looking for something that was an apparent hot commodity—a one-story home. I got lucky and landed in a neighborhood that had one left and snatched it up. The sales counselor noted that most people my age (she assumed I was in my 30s, so I'll take that as a win) preferred a two-story home for the larger living space and the potential views, so she was very curious as to why I was so set on a one-story. The truth was, I had been experiencing occasional discomfort when taking the stairs, attempting lunges, or even trying out the latest dance moves for quite some time. Considering that several members of my large extended family had already undergone at least one knee replacement surgery, I, as someone who tends to plan ahead, saw myself getting ready for what seemed inevitable—my own knee replacement surgery by the time I reached 60.

The reality of my physical condition became even more apparent a few months later during the pandemic. At the time, I was working in tech at Dropbox. As one of the first companies to announce permanent work-from-home, they'd boosted an already impressive list of employee benefits and perks that allowed me to set up the home office of my dreams. I loved being able to work from home, but the monotony of a daily routine that only included going between my bedroom, my kitchen, and my home office did little for my overall physical health. Two years later the world was getting back to its new normal, however, I found myself not only with more knee pain, but hip pain, and the inability to wear high heels or sit cross-legged was added to the bunch. This was unacceptable and I vowed to do something about it.

So, who am I to guide you through this journey? I'm not an expert, just a woman determined to reclaim a life filled with quality and vitality. I've immersed myself in research, consulted with various professionals, and dedicated hours to understanding knee pain causes and remedies. What you'll find in this book is not a claim of expertise but an authentic sharing of what works for me—knowledge that I believe can be your starting point toward optimal health.

I understand the discomfort of feeling unable to participate fully in fitness classes. I too have spent time with friends joking—but not joking— about our bad knees. I also find myself ashamed to try certain excursions when traveling for fear I won't be able to do it. We've all had excuses and ladies let me tell you, it's time to discard them. Together, we'll explore a new path—one that defies the notion that fitness goals are impossible for those with knee challenges.

In the bustling rhythm of modern life, where time is often our scarcest resource, the pursuit of fitness can feel like an unattainable goal—especially for the many incredible women facing the challenge of weak or bad knees. *Quick Home Workouts for Women with Bad Knees* isn't just a fitness guide; it's a roadmap to holistic well-being. In just 15 minutes a day, we'll reshape your perspective on fitness, introducing knee-friendly exercises that empower you to transcend limitations. This book is more than a collection of workouts; it's a promise that you can redefine what's possible for your health.

Embark on this journey with me, not as an expert, but as a companion on the path to well-being. Let's debunk the myth that effective workouts demand hours of dedication. Your fitness goals are within reach, and this book is your guide to revitalizing your life—one knee-friendly workout at a time.

2

Knee Pain: A Common Challenge

The knee, our body's largest joint and a cornerstone of our mobility, often becomes a source of discomfort. Knee pain affects approximately 1 in 4 adults, marking a significant and growing concern in our modern world. The prevalence of knee pain has surged by almost 65% over the past two decades, resulting in nearly 4 million primary care visits annually. This chapter sheds light on the importance of knee health for women—a crucial yet often overlooked aspect of overall well-being.

For us girls, knee pain is a multifaceted issue, influenced by anatomy, lifestyle, and specific health conditions. Factors such as wider hips, hormonal changes, and increased stress on the knees contribute to the vulnerability we face. Common symptoms of knee discomfort are pain, swelling, redness, weakness, stiffness, and locking.

Understanding the root cause of knee pain is crucial before addressing its symptoms. Various factors, such as aging, injuries, arthritis, overuse, and lack of activity, contribute to knee discomfort. Seeking professional guidance through medical history reviews, physical examinations, and imaging tests like X-rays and MRIs ensures an accurate diagnosis.

Treatment approaches vary, ranging from conservative measures like R.I.C.E (Rest, Ice, Compression, Elevation), herbal remedies, and Tai Chi, to physical therapy and surgical interventions for severe cases. However, our focus in this book centers on the empowering role of exercise as a conservative measure.

Contrary to the instinct to avoid exercise for fear of worsening knee pain, engaging in knee-friendly exercises is vital for averting further decline. In reality, these exercises play a crucial role in fortifying weakened knees. Comprehensive knee-strengthening routines focus on enhancing the quadriceps, hamstrings, glutes, and calves—the muscles surrounding the knee. This targeted approach not only improves knee strength but also enhances joint stability and provides essential support. Embracing low-impact activities like swimming, cycling, and modified strength training not only safeguards joint health but also contributes to overall fitness.

Weakened knees can have a ripple effect on the entire body, affecting mobility, stability, and contributing to pain in various areas. From strained hips to compromised balance, reduced cardiovascular fitness, and a diminished quality of life, the repercussions are extensive. Lifestyle adjustments are key contributors to sustained knee health. Maintaining a healthy weight alleviates stress on the knees, making a significant impact on existing conditions. Supportive footwear enhances joint stability, and incorporating regular stretching and warm-ups before exercise reduces the risk of injury. By embracing knee-friendly exercises and prioritizing joint health, women can embark on a journey towards pain-free movement and active living.

3

Workout Methods

So, confession time: I'm not exactly BFFs with working out. Hate might be a strong word, but let's just say I'm more on the apathetic side. It's like brushing my teeth—you won't catch me loving it, but I do it twice a day anyway.

But here's the real scoop—it took me a hot minute to figure out that fitness isn't one-size-fits-all. Sure, our goals might look similar, but our journeys? Totally unique. The magic formula? Finding activities that don't make you want to hit the snooze button on your workout.

It's all about turning exercise from a chore to a fulfilling part of your routine. Whether it's dancing, hiking, yoga (even if it's not my jam), or any other activity that floats your boat, falling in love with what you do ensures that fitness becomes a lifelong adventure, not a short-term obligation.

As for me, I've found my happy place to be a mix of strength training, Pilates, stretching, and a dash of cardio.

Strength Training: Think building muscle, boosting metabolism, and supporting joint stability. Whether it's lifting weights, rocking resistance bands, or crushing bodyweight exercises, focus on non-weight-bearing muscle groups like your upper body and core for heavier weights and save lighter to no weights for lower body exercises. And hey, proper form is the secret sauce.

Pilates: It's my go-to low-impact superstar, working on that core strength, flexibility, and overall body goodness. Unlike yoga, it lets me respond to my body's constant need to be on the move and keeps me in the zone.

Stretching: Flexibility is the name of the game here. Stretching eases muscle tension, boosts joint mobility, and keeps everything moving smoothly. Opt for gentle stretches that don't throw shade at your knees—no deep knee bends, just easy-breezy moves.

Cardio: Let's not forget the heartbeat accelerator! Cardio keeps things lively, gets your blood pumping, and boosts overall endurance. It's all about choosing activities that are gentle on the joints such as swimming, walking, cycling, rowing, and dancing. Whether it's a brisk walk, a jog, or even a dance session, cardio adds that extra zing to your routine.

Quick heads up, though: Before you dive into any exercise, especially if your knees are in the mix, a chat with a healthcare professional or a fitness guru is a smart move. They'll make sure your fitness journey is all about safety and suits your unique needs.

4

The Power of Short Workouts

In the hustle of our daily lives, finding time for workouts can feel like an Olympic feat, especially for us ladies kickstarting our fitness journey. Now, your friend might be pushing you to embrace the "more is better" philosophy, but recently a different path has emerged. The prevalent belief that more exercise is always better is being challenged by recent research, highlighting the potential drawbacks of prolonged and intense workouts, such as overuse injuries and chronic inflammation.

Contrary to the misconception that longer durations equate to better results, studies indicate that shorter, focused workouts offer tangible health benefits. Even brief, intense bursts of exercise, like climbing stairs or sprinting, are associated with positive outcomes for muscle building and cardiovascular health. The emphasis here is on intensity rather than duration, redefining the landscape of effective exercise.

For beginners, particularly women venturing into fitness or managing knee pain, the 15-minute workout emerges as an accessible and less intimidating gateway. It offers a manageable starting point, fostering a routine without overwhelming you. The beauty of these short sessions lies in the gentle progression, ensuring you build strength and stamina at your own pace, minimizing the risk of exacerbating knee pain.

Consistency takes precedence over intensity, with the 15-minute sessions proving to be more feasible for busy schedules. Regular, shorter workouts surpass sporadic, lengthy sessions, significantly contributing to overall health. Tailoring these brief routines to focus on specific movements, such as low-impact exercises or joint-friendly activities, meets the unique needs of women with knee pain, facilitating targeted strengthening without undue stress.

Beyond physical benefits, short bursts of exercise positively impact mental well-being. The release of endorphins during a quick 15-minute session acts as a powerful mood enhancer, contributing to reduced stress and improved mood and energy levels. The versatility of these workouts, whether through brisk walks, bodyweight exercises, or gentle stretching, allows for customization based on individual preferences and fitness levels.

In essence, the magic of 15-minute workouts lies not in their duration but in their consistency, adaptability, and ability to cater to individual needs. For women embarking on their fitness journey or managing knee pain, these short sessions stand as a catalyst for a transformative path toward improved health and overall well-being. Get ready to crush it in just 15 minutes!

5

The Reward: Stability, Strength, and Vitality

Embarking on knee-friendly workouts is a transformative journey that extends far beyond preserving joint health. These exercises, tailored to support and strengthen the knees, play a pivotal role in enhancing stability, facilitating weight loss, building strength, and boosting energy levels.

Improved Stability: Knee-friendly workouts often incorporate exercises that enhance overall stability. Focus on movements that engage the core, lower body, and stabilizing muscles around the knees. Strengthening these areas contributes to better balance and reduced risk of falls or injuries.

Facilitates Weight Loss: Engaging in knee-friendly exercises facilitates weight loss by creating a sustainable approach to physical activity. By minimizing the impact on joints, individuals can maintain consistent workouts, burning calories and contributing to a healthy weight. It's important to note, that while spending 15 minutes on your workout can really help to enhance and sustain muscle strength, if shedding some pounds is your objective, you'll want to add more time to your exercise routine. The goal is to work your way up to a 30-minute session, throw in some cardio, and most importantly, make sure you're keeping tabs on your eating habits and diet.

Enhanced Strength: Knee-friendly workouts emphasize strengthening the muscles surrounding the knees without placing excessive stress on the joints. This targeted approach enhances muscle endurance, flexibility, and joint support, fostering overall strength and resilience.

Energy Boost: Regular, knee-friendly exercises stimulate the cardiovascular system, promoting better circulation and oxygenation of tissues. This, in turn, results in an energy boost. Short, low-impact workouts can be particularly effective in combating fatigue and enhancing vitality.

Joint Health Preservation: Knee-friendly workouts are designed to prioritize joint health. By incorporating exercises that minimize impact and focus on controlled, deliberate movements, individuals can preserve the integrity of their knees. This proactive approach is essential for long-term joint health and mobility.

Increased Range of Motion: Knee-friendly exercises often involve dynamic stretches and movements that contribute to an increased range of motion. This not only supports joint health but also enhances flexibility, making daily activities more comfortable and efficient.

Boosts Mental Well-Being: Physical activity, especially knee-friendly workouts, releases endorphins—the body's natural mood boosters. Regular exercise has been linked to reduced stress, anxiety, and improved overall mental well-being, contributing to a positive outlook on life.

Adaptable to Varied Fitness Levels: Knee-friendly workouts are versatile and can be adapted to accommodate different fitness levels. Whether you're a beginner, recovering from an injury, or an advanced fitness enthusiast, these exercises provide a scalable and inclusive approach to physical activity.

Consistent Progression: Consistency is key in any fitness journey, and knee-friendly workouts facilitate a consistent approach to exercise. By avoiding excessive strain on the knees, individuals can maintain regularity in their workouts, ensuring steady progress over time.

Supports Long-Term Fitness Goals: Knee-friendly workouts are sustainable and supportive of long-term fitness goals. They create a foundation for a healthy and active lifestyle, allowing individuals to enjoy the benefits of exercise without compromising joint health.

In essence, knee-friendly workouts are a holistic approach to fitness, promoting stability, weight loss, strength, and sustained energy. By prioritizing joint health and incorporating tailored exercises, you can embark on a journey toward improved well-being and vitality.

6

Getting Started: A Guide to Success

For years, I'd been hearing about this health and wellness resort in St Lucia called The Body Holiday. Their motto, "Give us your body for a week and we'll give you back your mind," just sounded too good to pass up. So in 2022, after a rollercoaster of a year, I decided to take the plunge. And let me spill the tea—it lived up to every ounce of the hype!

Picture this: pristine beaches, perfect weather, and more dolphins than I thought I'd ever see in my life. The resort itself? A dream. Gorgeous rooms, mouthwatering healthy meals, top-notch entertainment, a daily lineup of mind-body classes, and the cherry on top— a body treatment every single day. I was officially hooked.

Now, here's where it gets interesting. While hanging out at the Ayurveda temple (fancy, right?), I decided to dive into the world of Doshas. According to Ayurveda, Doshas are the 'energy principles' that run the show in our bodies and minds. Each Dosha comes with its own set of qualities that influence everything from how you digest food to how you process emotions. Turns out, my main Dosha is Vata.

So, Vatas, we're the creative, dynamic, whirlwind types. Quick minds, but, you know, we might forget where we left our keys. The Ayurveda guru pointed out some signs that my Vata was a bit off-balance—tiredness, lack of focus, feeling anxious, and the struggle to catch those Zs. Bingo! That was me.

But fear not, the remedy was laid out simple. Three warm, well-cooked meals at the same time every day (no more hangry moments), daily downtime, regular exercise, and a consistent bedtime. As you can see the theme here is routine, routine, routine. According to my dosha, its the prescription for getting my groove back.

Embarking on a fitness journey requires thoughtful planning and a commitment to your well-being. Here's a guide on what you need to kickstart your workouts, stay motivated, and build a sustainable routine.

Set your intentions

Understanding your 'why' is the key to success with anything. Define clear and realistic goals, whether they're related to weight loss, muscle gain, improved cardiovascular health, or overall well-being. Break down long-term goals into smaller, achievable milestones for a sense of accomplishment. Understand the deeper motivations behind your fitness journey. Whether it's increased energy, stress relief, or improved self-esteem, a strong "why" can fuel your commitment.

Set up your home gym

You can definitely join a gym, but I've found that I'm more successful when I work out at home. Start with low-cost items like resistance bands, a yoga mat, and a stability ball. It's also helpful to have access to dumbbell(s) and kettlebell(s) for a basic home gym setup. I have blocked off half of my garage for my workouts. I have a small, but mighty collection of fitness equipment and tools in my garage gym.

- treadmill (courtesy of that tech job I spoke about in the introduction)
- set of adjustable dumbbells
- one adjustable kettlebell
- fitness/stability ball
- foam roller
- variety of resistance bands
- weight bench
- Pilates bar
- yoga blocks
- yoga mats
- knee pads

I'd really suggest getting yourself some adjustable dumbbells and kettlebells – you can grab them at Walmart, Target, Best Buy, or Amazon. They're not only space-savers but also a time-saver when you're hopping between exercises. Don't forget about knee pads – they're a game-changer for more comfy kneeling exercises. Apart from my garage gym setup, I've got a yoga mat, yoga blocks, and a Pilates bar in my family room. It's my go-to spot when I want to catch up on TV while breaking a sweat.

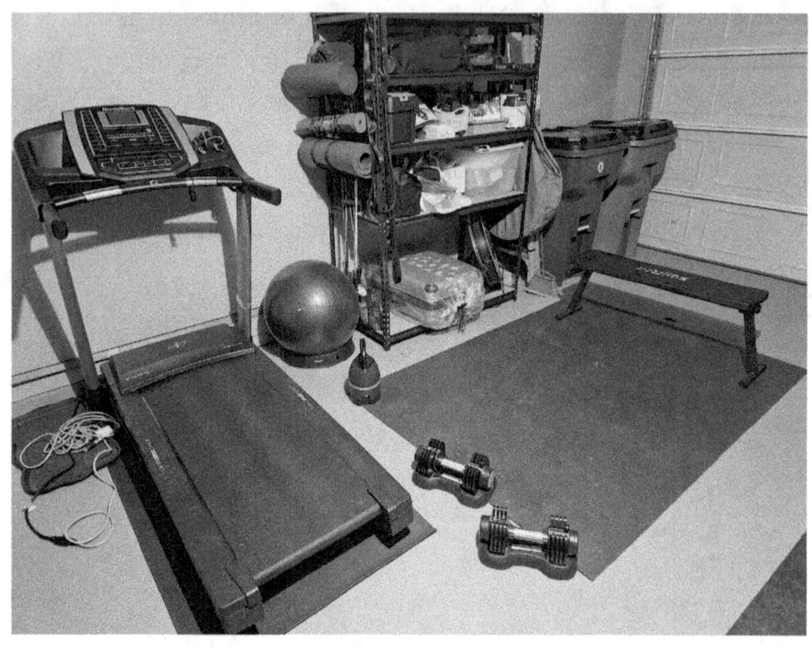

My home gym in my garage

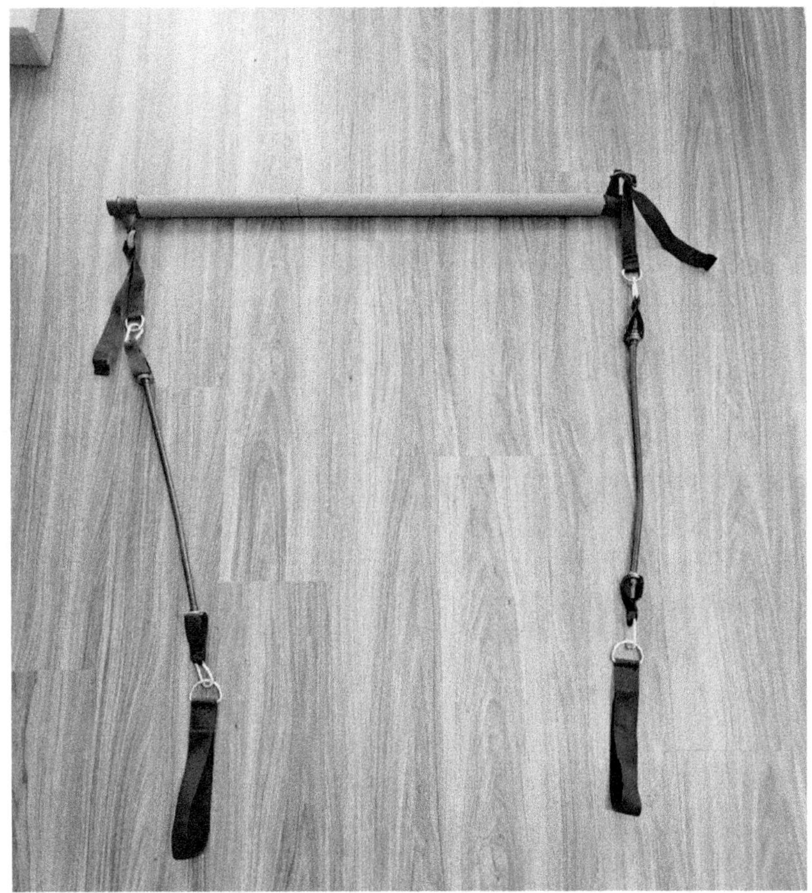

My movie companion, the Pilates bar

Planning your workouts

Since the workouts are only 15 minutes, I suggest working out 6 days a week. However, decide how many days per week you can commit to working out. Choose specific days and times that align with your schedule and energy levels. You can always adjust as you go. Here's what a sample week could look like:

Monday: Strength training (lower body/core)
Tuesday: Strength training (upper body)
Wednesday: Pilates (lower body/core)
Thursday: Pilates (upper body)
Friday: Rest day
Saturday: Strength training (total body) or rest day
Sunday: Cardio, stretching, or rest day

Take measurements and pics

Taking measurements and pictures before starting a new fitness regimen provides a comprehensive and personalized view of your starting point. It becomes a valuable tool for tracking progress, setting realistic goals, staying motivated, and making informed adjustments to your fitness plan along the way.

Try temptation bundling

Temptation bundling, a concept introduced by researcher Katie Milkman and her colleagues, aims to make mundane tasks more enjoyable by combining them with activities that bring instant gratification. The idea is simple: pair an activity you don't like with something you do enjoy. For instance, you might listen to music or check Instagram while running on the treadmill or engage in other less enjoyable tasks. The key is to allow yourself the "fun" activity only when coupled with the "not-so-fun" one. In a study led by Milkman, participants were given iPods with exclusive audio novels accessible only during workouts, resulting in increased gym attendance as it became linked with a pleasurable indulgence. This technique has been highly effective for me.

Do not skip the warm-up

Prioritize a proper warm-up to increase blood flow, prepare muscles and joints, and reduce the risk of injury. Dynamic stretches, light cardio, or bodyweight exercises help activate key muscle groups. I've included warm-up exercises in each workout routine. Believe me. Your knees will be much happier.

Make time for a cool-down

Allocate time for a cool-down session to gradually lower heart rate and prevent muscle stiffness. This is a great time to do static stretches as it enhances flexibility and improves range of motion. Cool-downs are also included in the workout routines.

Rest days and recovery

Plan rest days to allow your body to recover and prevent burnout. Adequate sleep, hydration, and nutrition are crucial components of recovery.

Avoiding injury

Listen to your body and avoid pushing yourself too hard, too soon and focus on proper form during exercises to prevent strain or injury. Gradually progress intensity and volume to allow your body to adapt.

Variety

I once had a personal trainer who gave me different exercises to do every day. I never performed the same exercise twice. While I appreciate the importance of variety, how will I know I improved with an exercise if I never repeat it?

Olympic lifting coach, Evelyn Valdez dispels the misconception that constant variation is universally beneficial. While acknowledging the significance of variety, she cautions against too frequent changes, emphasizing the need for consistent stress to foster improvement. She advocates for changing strength training exercises every 4-6 weeks while maintaining a handful of indicator exercises such as deadlifts or planks that you use to gauge your progress.

Remember, every fitness journey is unique, and progress takes time. Celebrate small victories, stay patient, and be adaptable in your approach. Whether you're working out at home or in a gym, the key is consistency and a commitment to your long-term health and well-being. If in doubt, consult with a fitness professional to tailor a program to your individual needs.

Ready to rock these workouts? Let's do this!

7

How-Tos: Knee Friendly Exercises

Here is a curated collection of exercises designed to strengthen and tone that will not only be kind to your joints but also invigorate your entire body. Each exercise is accompanied by images and instructions on how to perform them correctly to make sure you execute each movement with confidence. If additional guidance is needed to properly perform any of these exercises, a quick search on Google or YouTube will provide video demonstrations to guide you through each movement. Remember to listen to your body, modify exercises as needed, and enjoy your workout!

Warm-up Exercises

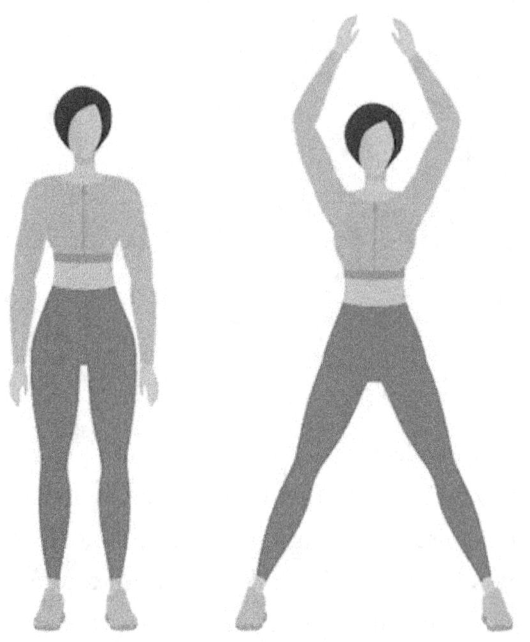

Jumping Jacks

- *Muscles Targeted*: Full body, especially legs, shoulders, and cardio-vascular system
- *Instructions:* Stand with feet together and arms relaxed at your sides. Jump, spreading legs and raising arms overhead. Return to the starting position.

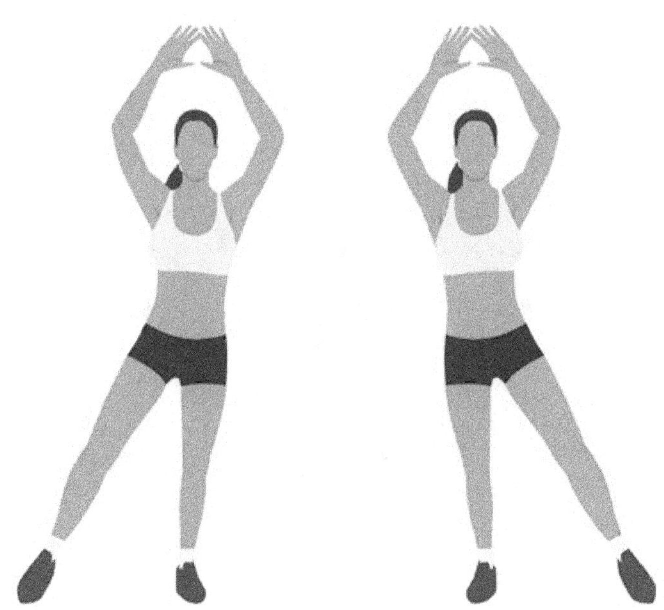

Jumping Jacks Modified

- *Muscles Targeted*: Full body, especially legs, shoulders, and cardio-vascular system
- *Instructions:* Stand with feet together and arms relaxed at your sides. Instead of the traditional jumping motion, step one foot out to the side while simultaneously raising your arms overhead. Return to the starting position and repeat on the other side.
- *Note:* This modified version reduces impact, making it gentler on

the joints while still providing a good cardiovascular workout

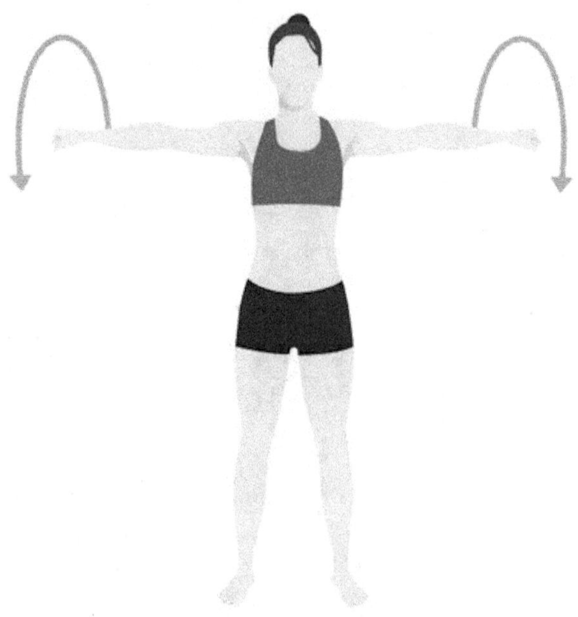

Arm Circles

- *Muscles Targeted:* Shoulders, arms
- *Instructions:* Extend arms to the sides. Make circular motions with your arms, clockwise and then counterclockwise.

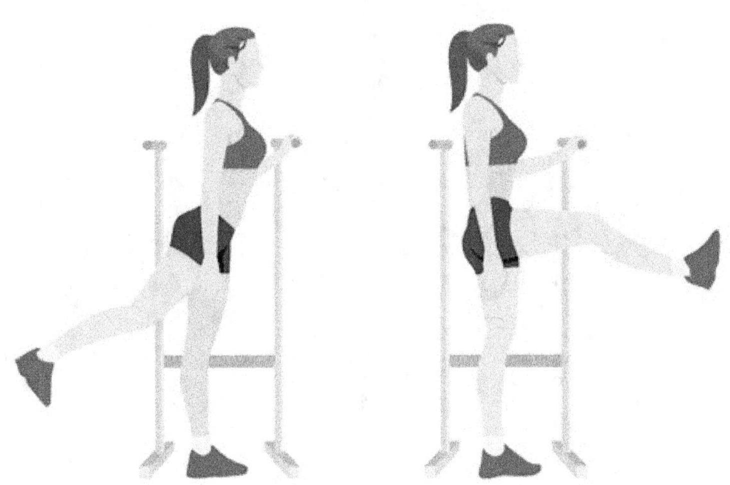

Forward Leg Swings

- *Muscles Targeted:* Hips, thighs
- *Instructions:* Hold onto a stable surface. Swing one leg forward and backward in a controlled motion.

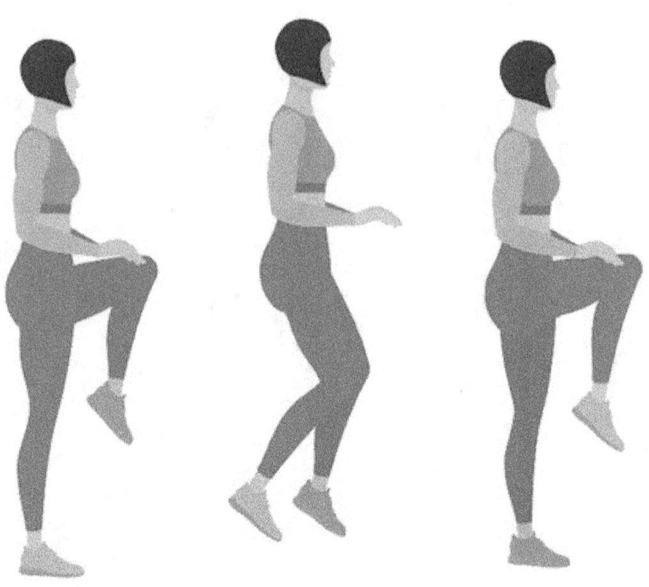

High Knees

- *Muscles Targeted:* Quadriceps, Hip Flexors
- *Instructions:* Stand with feet hip-width apart. Lift your knees toward your chest rapidly, alternating legs.
- *Notes:* Keep your back straight, engage your core, and land softly on the balls of your feet.

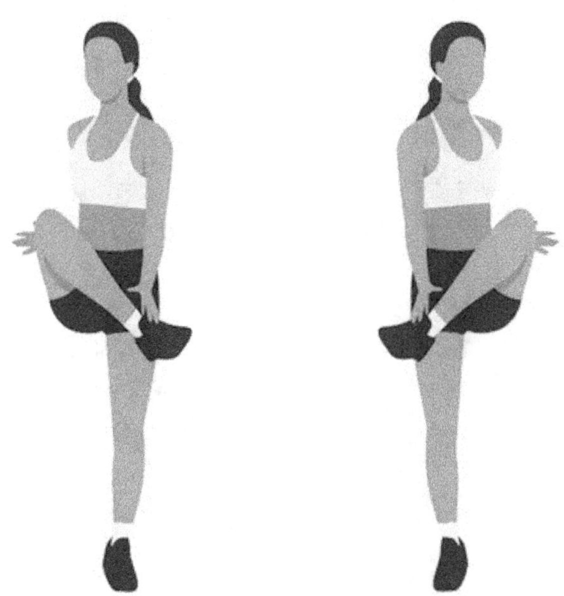

Fingertip-to-Toe Touches

- *Muscles Targeted:* Hamstrings, Obliques, Core
- *Instructions:* Stand with feet shoulder-width apart. Bring one foot up to touch the fingertips of your opposite hand. Alternate sides.
- *Notes:* Keep your hips facing forward and move in a controlled manner.

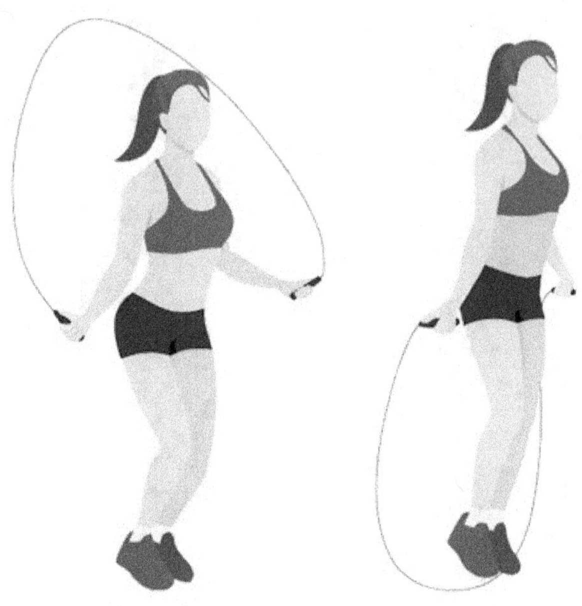

Jump Rope (real or imaginary)

- *Muscles Targeted:* Full Body (Cardiovascular)
- *Instructions:* Jump a rope or mimic the motion of jumping rope, landing softly on the balls of your feet.
- *Notes:* Maintain a steady pace and engage your arms as if holding a rope.

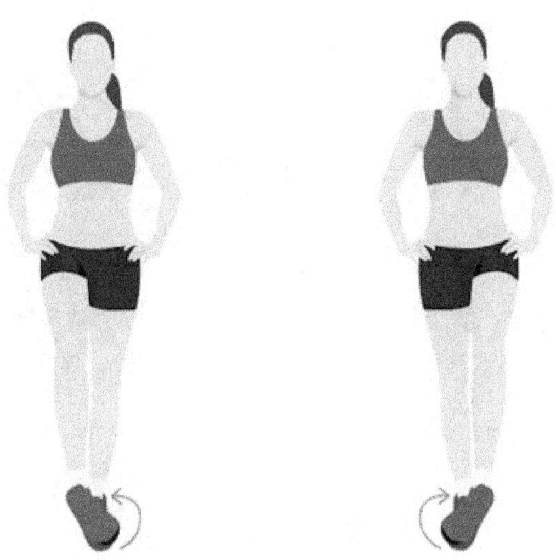

Ankle Circles

- *Muscles Targeted:* Ankle Joint
- *Instructions:* Standing, lift one foot and rotate your ankle clockwise, then counterclockwise. Repeat on the other foot.
- *Notes:* Perform gentle circles and focus on flexibility.

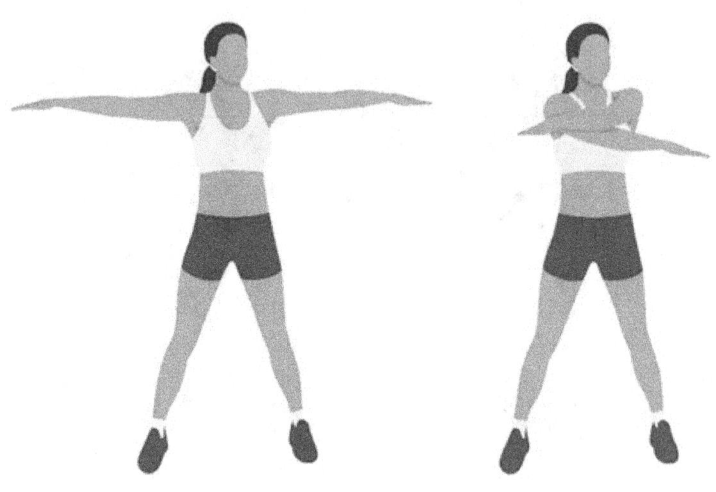

Arm Swings

- *Muscles Targeted:* Shoulders, Arms
- *Instructions:* Start with your arms straight out to the side and swing them in a crisscross fashion in front of your body.
- *Tips:* Gradually increase the range of motion as your muscles warm up.

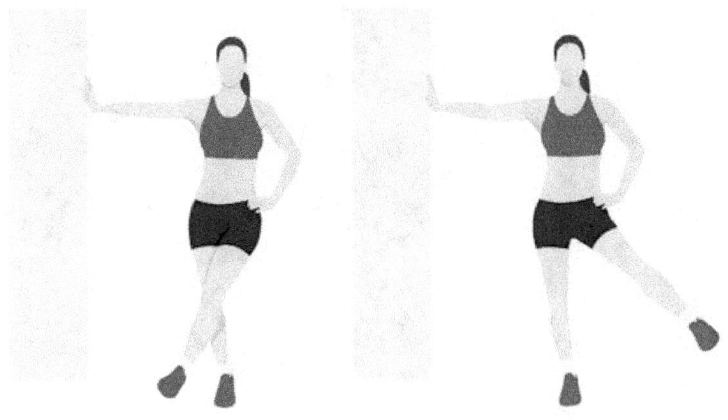

Lateral Leg Swings

- *Muscles Targeted:* Hip flexors, quadriceps
- *Instructions:* Stand beside a support and swing one leg from side to side keeping it straight. Switch legs.

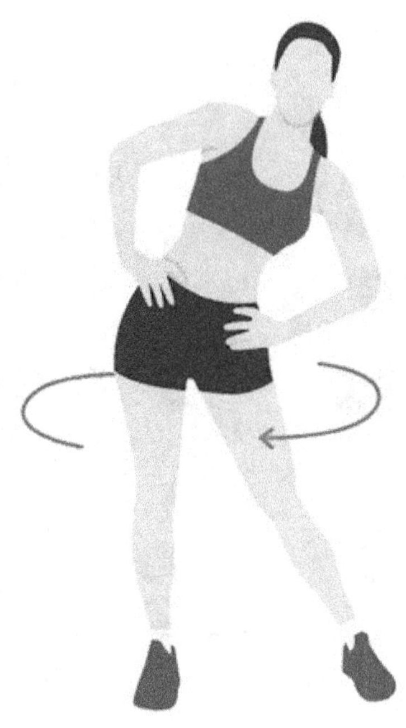

Hip Circles

- *Muscles Targeted:* Hips, lower back
- *Instructions:* Stand with feet shoulder-width apart and hands on hips. Circle hips clockwise. Circle hips counterclockwise.

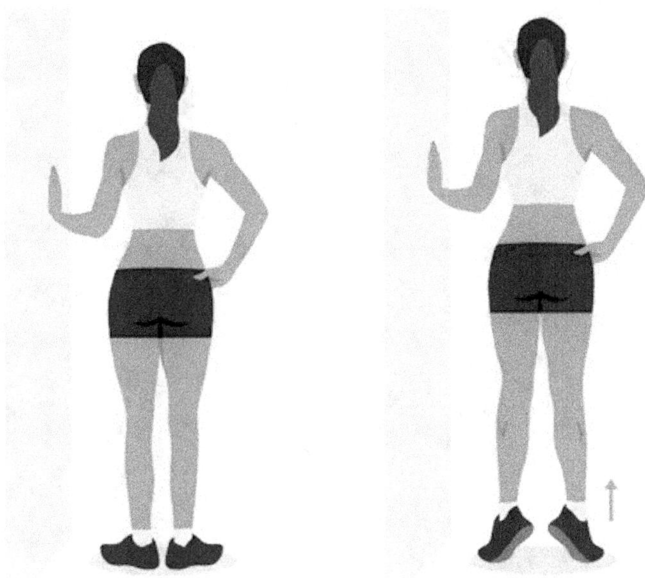

Calf Raises

- *Muscles Targeted:* Calves
- *Instructions:* Stand on a flat surface and stand beside a support. Lift heels off the ground by pushing through the balls of your feet. Lower and repeat.

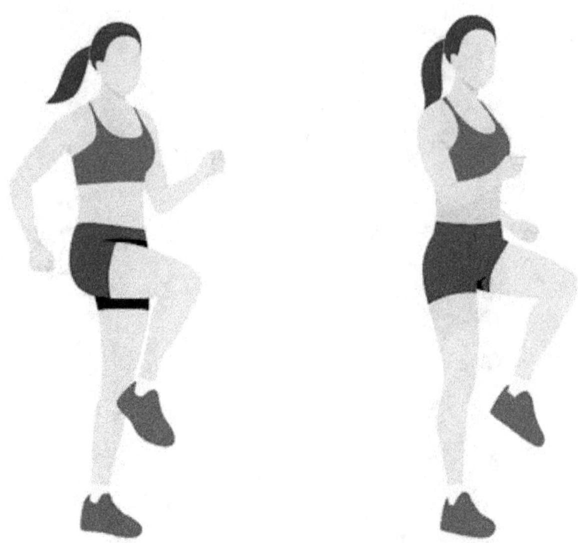

March in Place

- *Muscles Targeted:* Cardiovascular system, leg muscles.
- *Instructions:* Lift your knees alternatively, mimicking a marching motion.

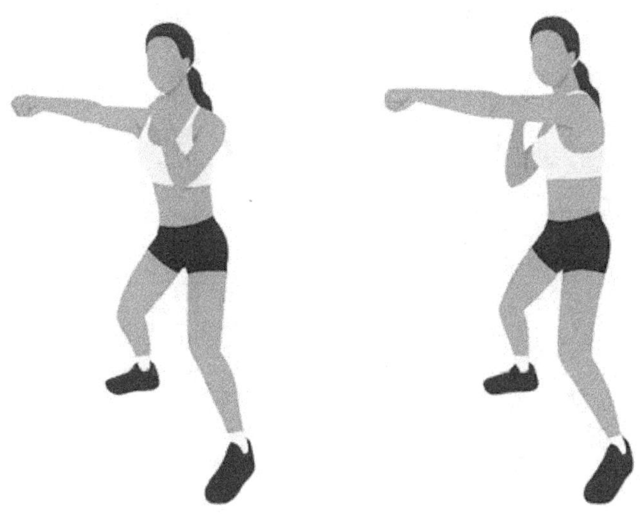

Jab-Cross

- *Muscles Targeted:* Quadriceps, hamstrings, glutes, core, shoulders
- *Instructions:* Stand with feet shoulder-width apart with a bend in your knee almost in a half squat. Jab with one fist, followed by a cross with the other.

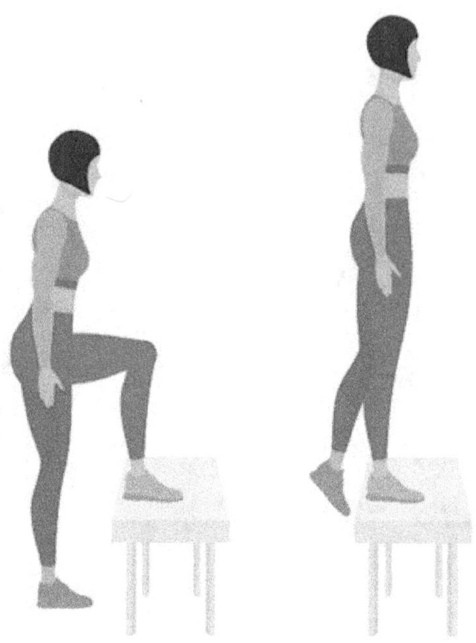

Step-Ups

- *Muscles Targeted:* Quadriceps, hamstrings, glutes
- *Instructions:* Use a sturdy bench or step. Step up with your right foot, then bring the left foot up. Step down with the right foot, followed by the left. Repeat alternating leading legs.

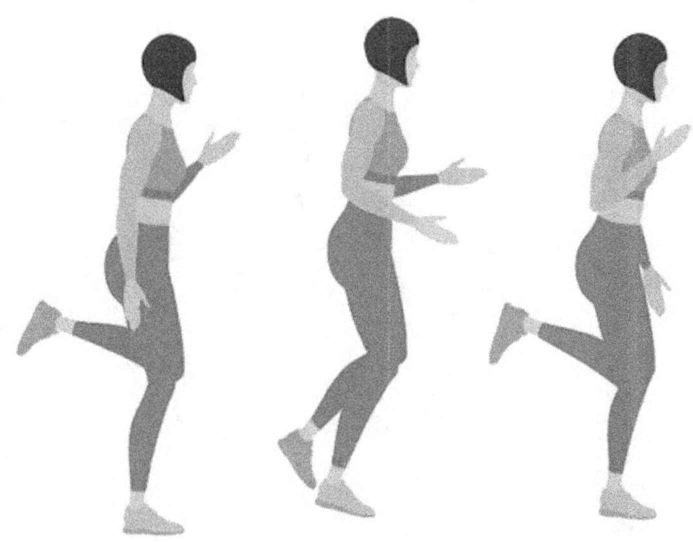

Butt Kicks

- *Muscles Targeted:* Hamstrings, glutes
- *Instructions:* Stand with feet hip-width apart and kick your heel toward your glutes. Alternate sides.

Full Body/Core Exercises

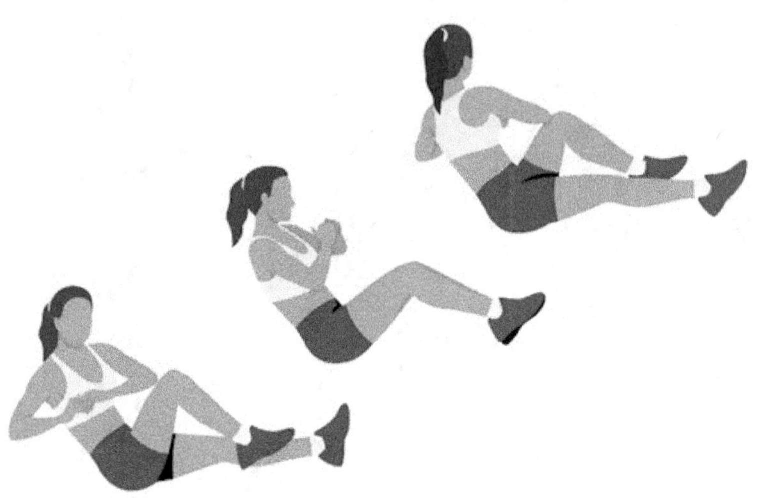

Bicycle Crunches

- *Muscles Targeted:* Abdominals, obliques
- *Instructions:* Lie on your back. Hinge at the waist and bring one knee toward the opposite elbow while extending the other leg.

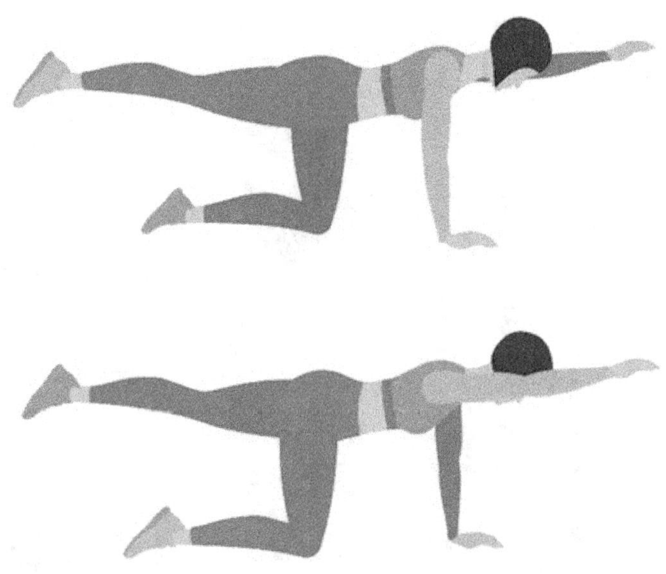

Bird-Dogs

- *Muscles Targeted:* Core, Lower Back
- *Instructions:* Start on hands and knees, extend one arm and the opposite leg simultaneously. Repeat in same direction before repeating on the other side.

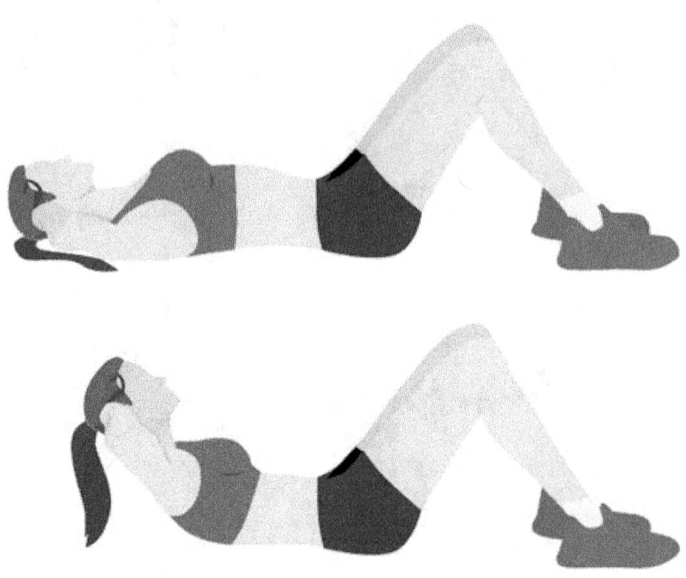

Crunches

- *Muscles Targeted:* Abdominals
- *Instructions:* Lie on your back with knees bent and hands behind your head. Lift your shoulders off the ground, engaging your core. Return to the starting position.

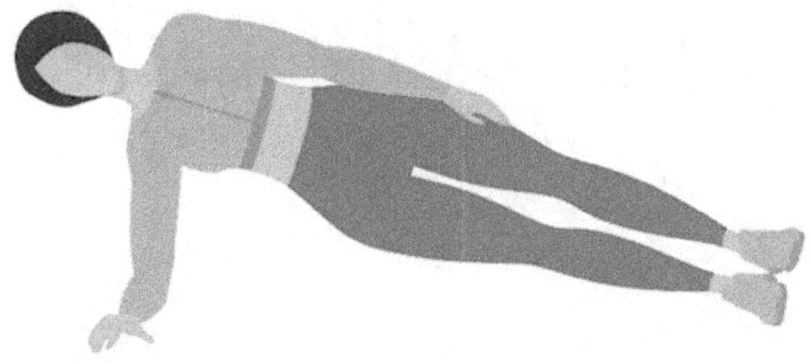

Side Plank

- *Muscles Targeted:* Core, obliques, shoulders
- *Instructions:* Lying on your side, push up on your elbow into a side plank position and hold. Switch sides.

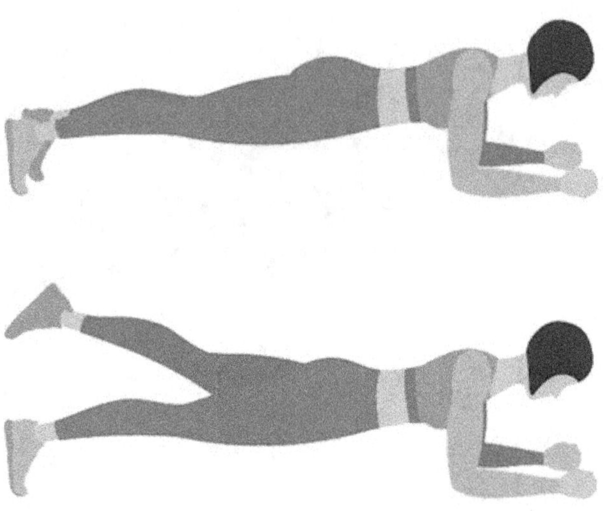

Plank with Leg Lifts

- *Muscles Targeted:* Core, shoulders, glutes
- *Instructions:* Face down on the ground and rest your weight on your elbows and your toes. Lift one leg at a time, keeping your spine straight and your core engaged.

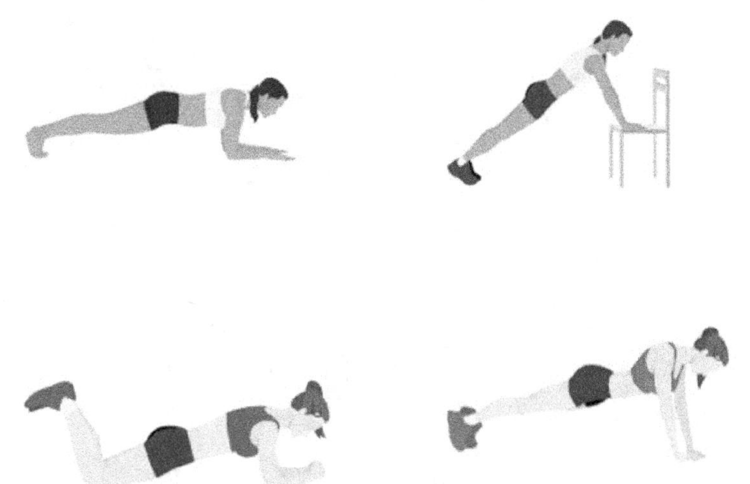

Top left: forearm plank; top right: chair plank; bottom left: forearm plank on knees; bottom right: plank

Plank Variations

- *Muscles Targeted:* Core, shoulders, back
- *Instructions (forearm):* From all fours, get in one of the plank positions above. Keep your body in a straight line and hold engaging your core.

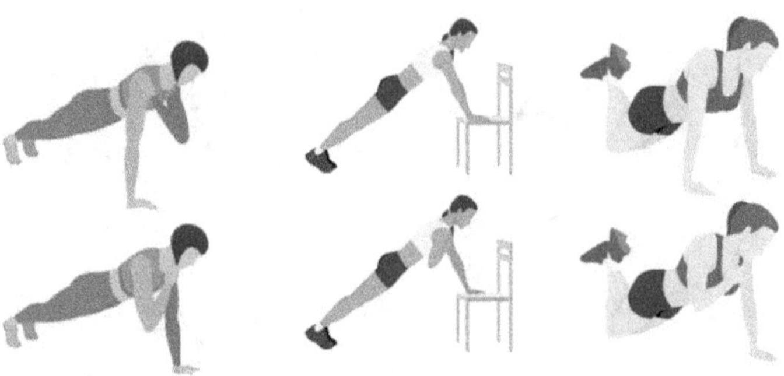

Left: plank on toes; middle: chair plank; right: plank on knees

Plank with Shoulder Taps

- *Muscles Targeted:* Core, Shoulders
- *Instructions:* Get in a plank position with legs extended, on your knees, or inclined from a chair. Tap your shoulders with the opposite hand.

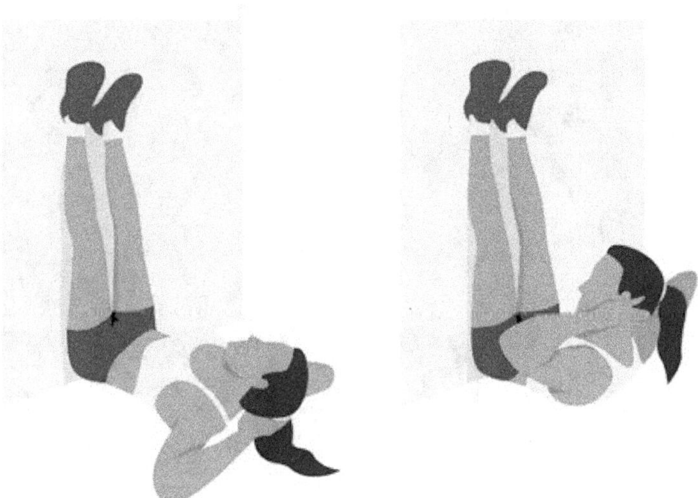

Leg Up the Wall Crunch

- *Muscles Targeted:* Abdominals
- *Instructions:* Lie on your back and extend your legs up the wall. Lift your shoulders off the floor halfway and lower it. Repeat.

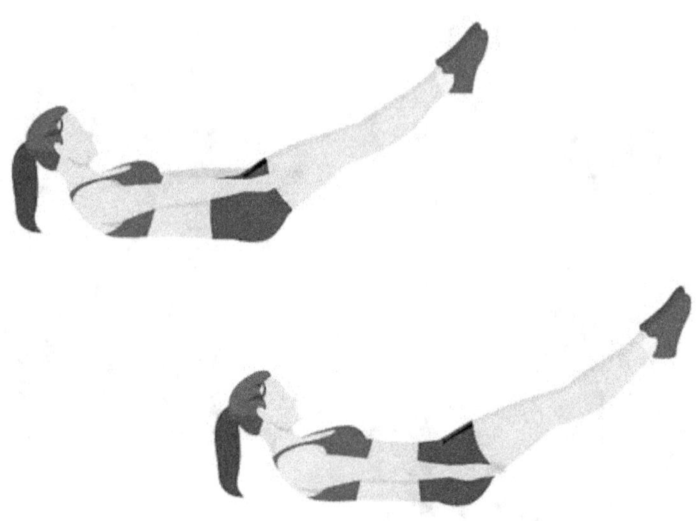

Pilates Hundred

- *Muscles Targeted:* Abdominals, Cardiovascular
- *Instructions:* Lie on your back. Lift your legs or your knees. Pump your arms up and down while inhaling for 5 counts and exhaling for 5 counts.

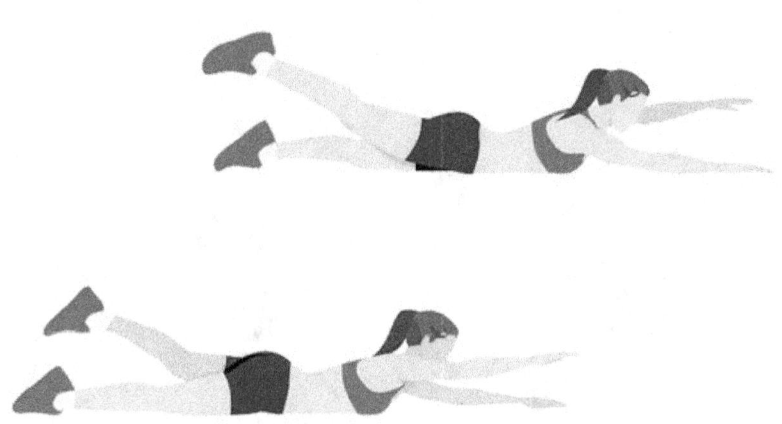

Pilates Swimming

- *Muscles Targeted:* Core, lower back, glutes
- *Instructions:* Lie face down with your arms and legs fully extended and straight. Lift your right arm and left leg simultaneously off the ground. Lower them to the ground and alternate sides.
- *Notes:* Keep your gaze towards the mat to maintain a neutral neck position. Engage your glutes to support your leg lifts.

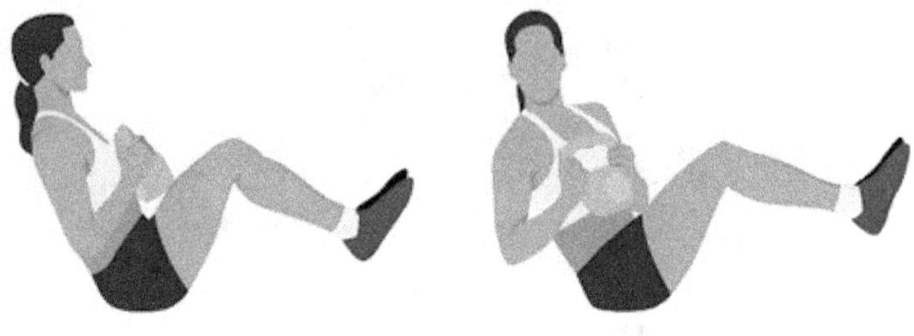

Russian Twists

- *Muscles Targeted:* Core, obliques
- *Instructions:* Sit on the floor with your knees bent and lean back slightly. Hold a kettlebell or your hands together. Twist your torso to the right, then to the left, tapping the ground beside you.

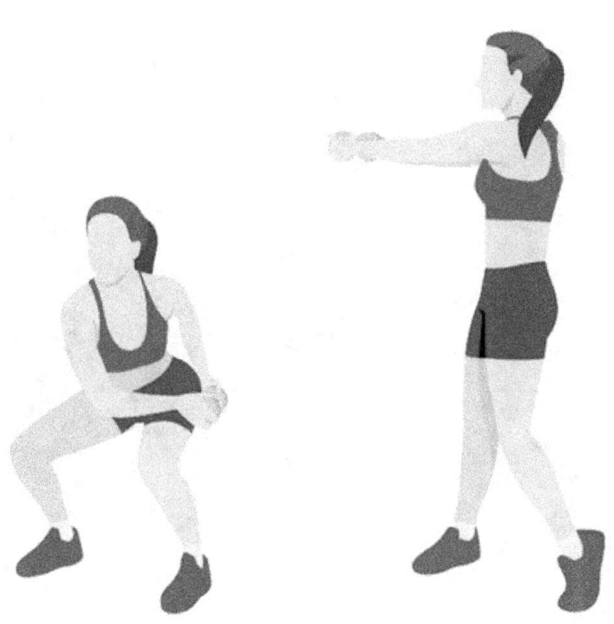

Wood Chops

- *Muscles Targeted*: Core, obliques, shoulders
- *Instructions:* Stand with feet shoulder-width apart, holding a kettlebell with both hands. Rotate your torso and chop the kettlebell diagonally across your body. Return to the starting position and repeat on the other side.

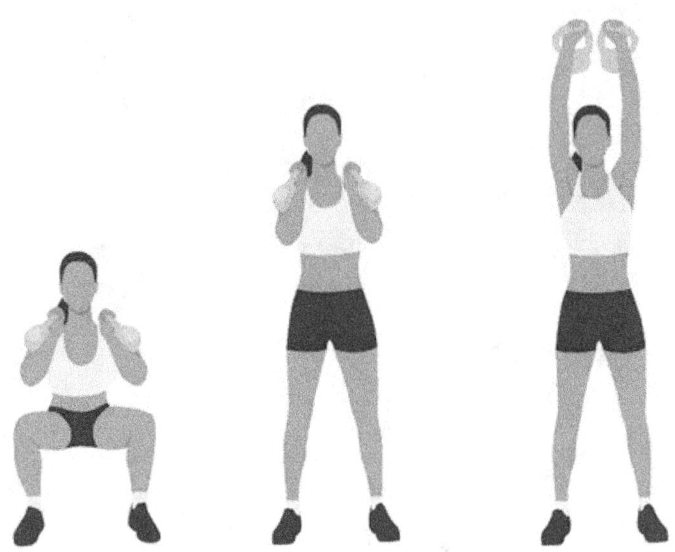

Goblet Squat to Overhead Press

- *Muscles Targeted:* Quads, Glutes, Shoulders
- *Instructions:* Hold a kettlebell close to your chest, squat, then press the kettlebell overhead as you stand.
- *Notes:* This can be done using a single kettlebell or two kettlebells. Keep your back straight and engage your core throughout.

Upper Body/Core Exercises

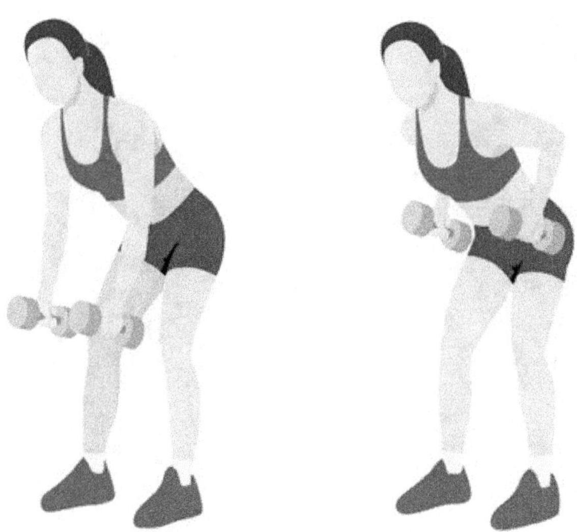

Bent-Over Rows with Dumbbells (or kettlebells)

- *Muscles Targeted:* Upper back, lats, biceps
- *Instructions:* Hinge at your hips, keeping back straight. Start with the dumbbells out in front of you, then pull them to your chest,

squeezing your shoulder blades.

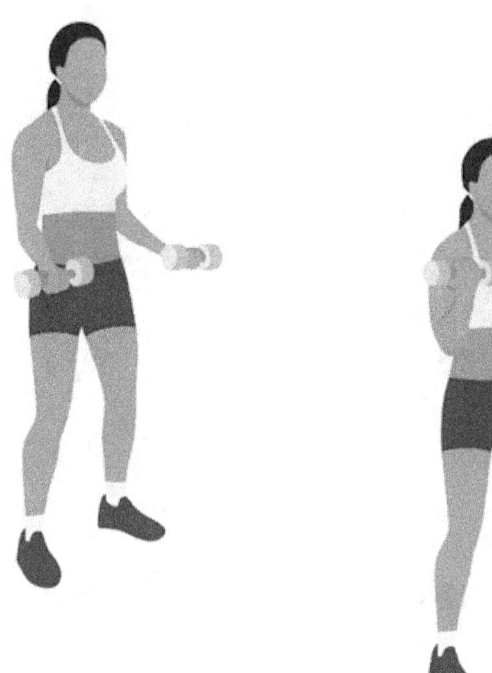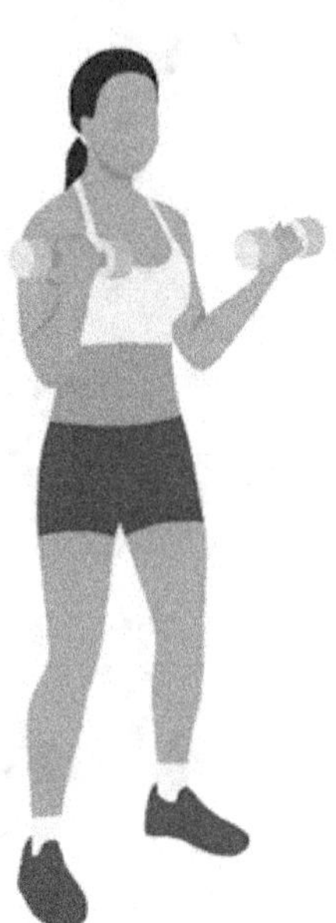

Bicep Curls with Dumbbells (or kettlebells or resistance bands)

- *Muscles Targeted:* Biceps
- *Instructions:* Hold dumbbells by your sides with your palms facing outward. Curl weights towards your shoulders.

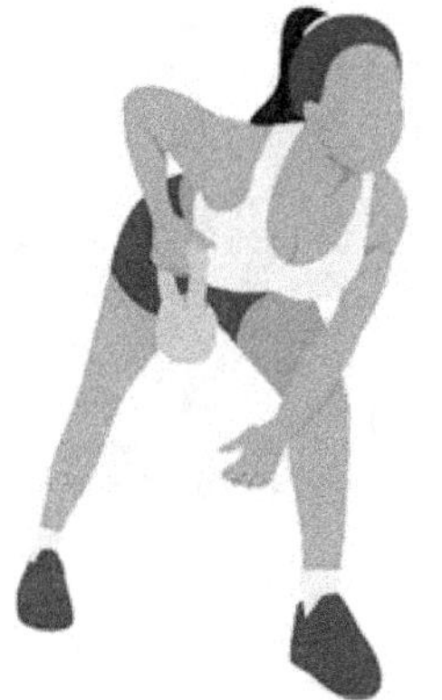 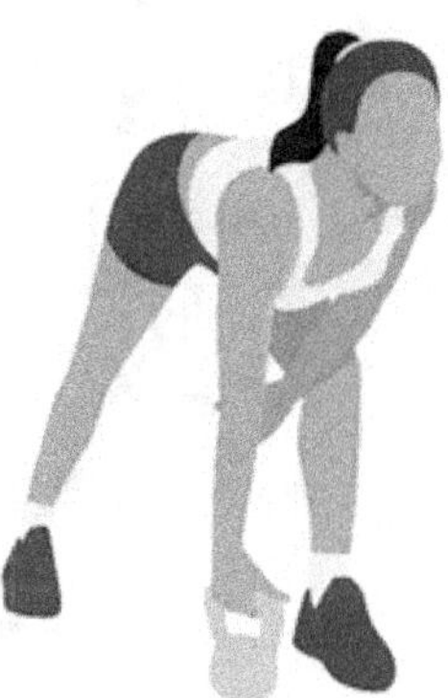

Bent-Over One-Arm Row with Kettlebell (or dumbbell):

- *Muscles Targeted:* Lats, Rhomboids, Biceps
- *Instructions:* Hinge at your hips, keep your back flat, and bend your arm at the elbow to row the kettlebell to your side.
- *Tips:* Keep your core engaged, and don't rush the movement.

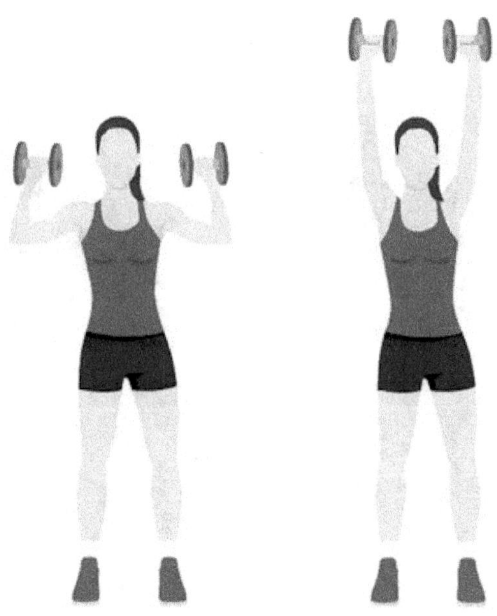

Overhead Press

- *Muscles Targeted:* Chest, shoulders, triceps
- *Instructions:* Sit or stand with dumbbells in hand. Press the dumbbells upward, extending your arms fully.

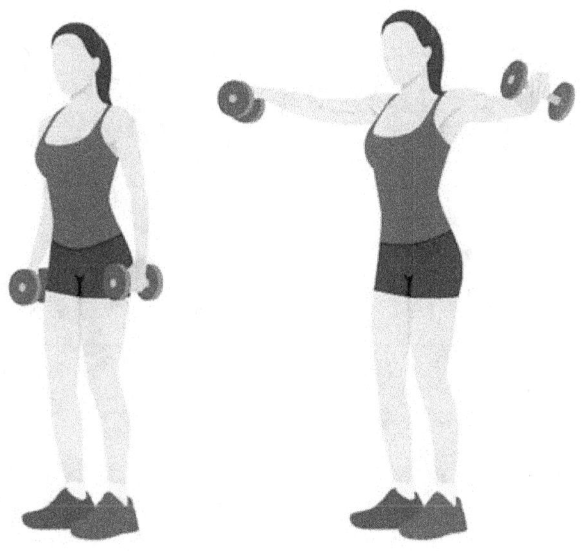

Lateral Arm Raises

- *Muscles Targeted:* Shoulders (lateral deltoids)
- *Instructions:* Stand with dumbbells at your sides. Lift the dumbbells out to the sides, keeping a slight bend in your elbows.

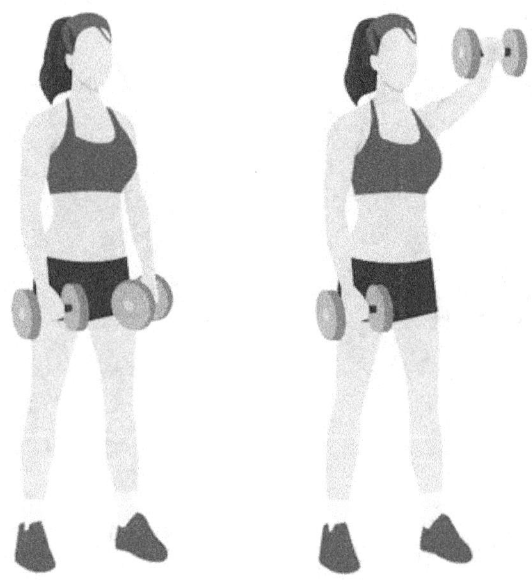

Front Arm Raise

- *Muscles Targeted:* Front deltoids (shoulders)
- *Instructions:* Stand with a dumbbell in each hand. With your palms facing your thighs, fully extend your arms directly in front of you until they reach shoulder height. Lower the dumbbells.

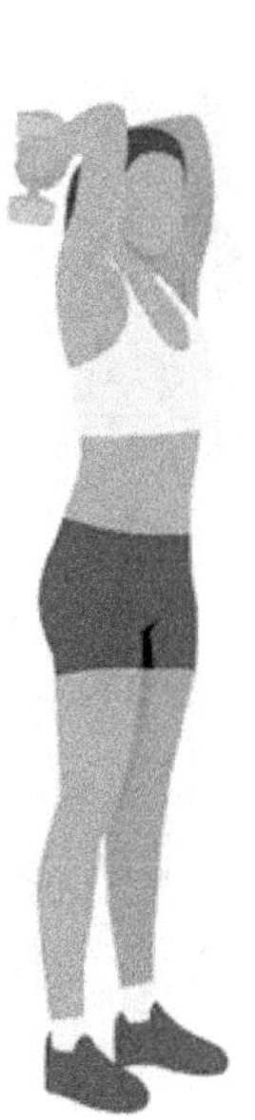
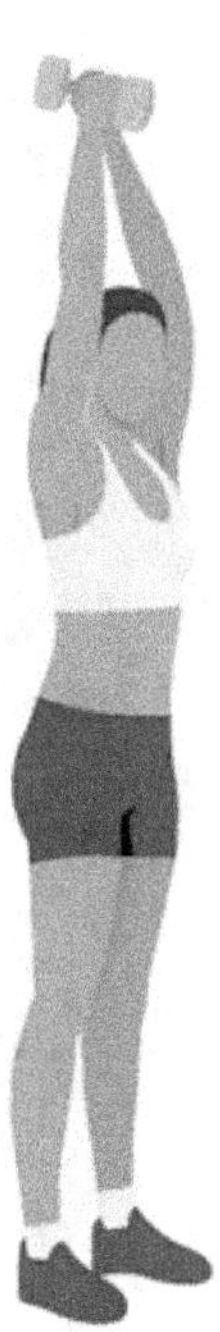

Tricep Extensions

- *Muscles Targeted:* Triceps
- *Instructions:* Hold a dumbbell overhead with both hands. Lower the dumbbell behind your head by bending your elbows.

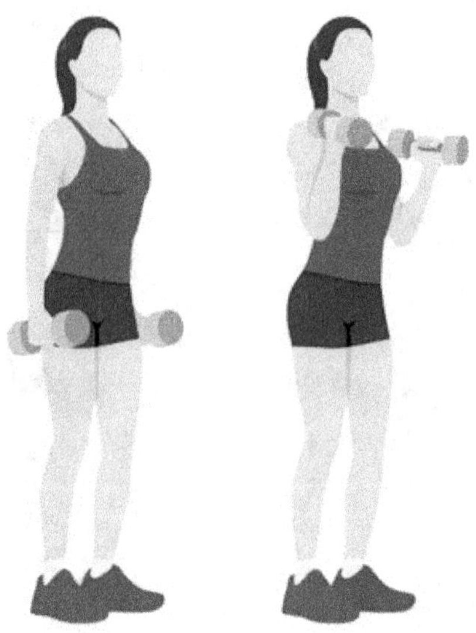

Hammer Grip Curls

- *Muscles Targeted*: Biceps
- *Instructions:* Hold a dumbbell in each hand with a neutral grip (palms facing each other) and curl the weights toward your shoulders. Lower to starting position.

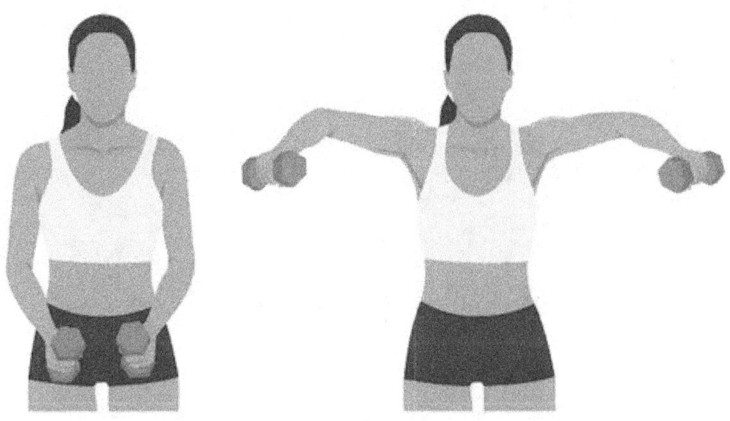

Lateral Side Shoulder Raises

- *Muscles Targeted*: Back, shoulders
- *Instructions:* Stand with feet shoulder-width apart, holding a dumbbell in each hand by your sides with a neutral grip and a slight bend in your elbow (palms facing your body). In a controlled motion, lift both arms directly to the sides until they reach shoulder height. Lower the dumbbells.

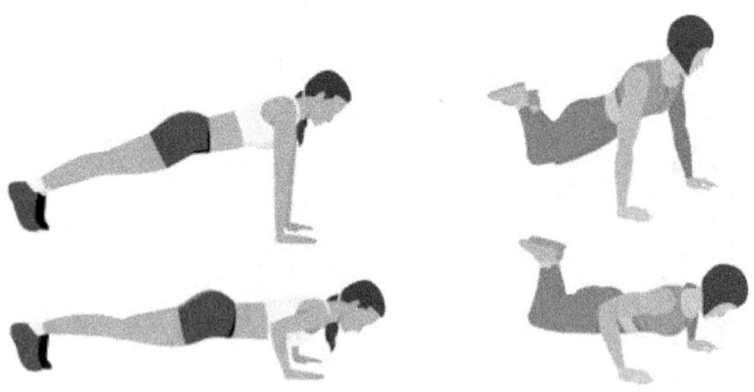

Left: standard push-up; right: modified push-up on knees

Push-ups

- *Muscles Targeted:* Chest, Shoulders, Triceps
- Reps/Sets: 12 reps, 3 sets
- Instructions: Get into a plank position with your toes or your knees on the ground. Lower your chest toward the floor and push back up.

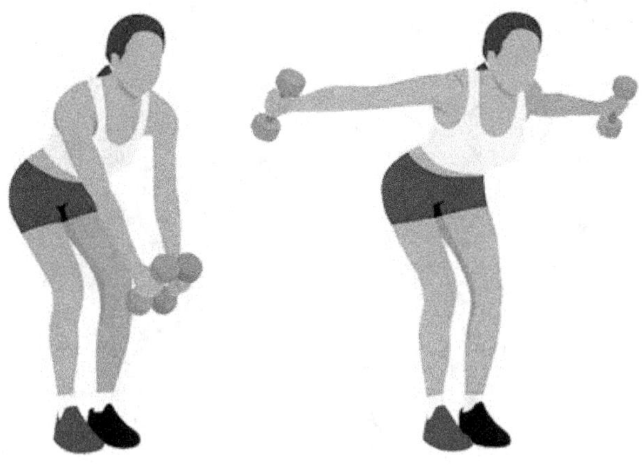

Reverse Fly

Muscles Targeted: Upper Back, Shoulders

Instructions: Hold a dumbbell in each hand, bend forward at the hips, and lift the weights to the side. Lower to the starting position.

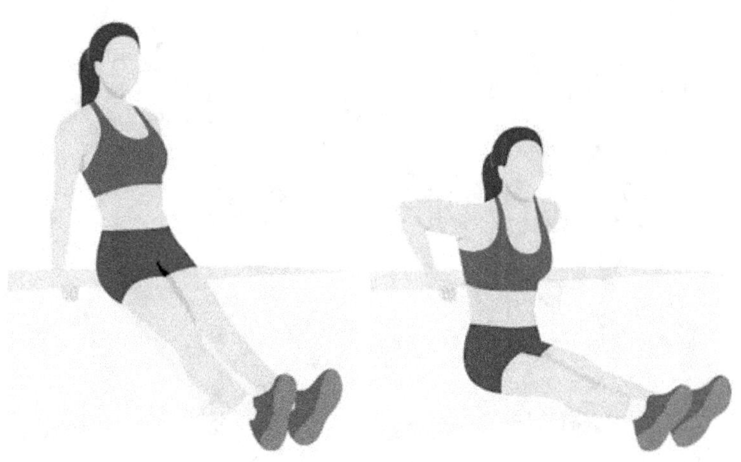

Tricep Dips

- *Muscles Targeted:* Triceps, Shoulders, Chest
- *Instructions:* Using parallel bars or the edge of a sturdy chair, lower your body by bending your elbows, then push back up.

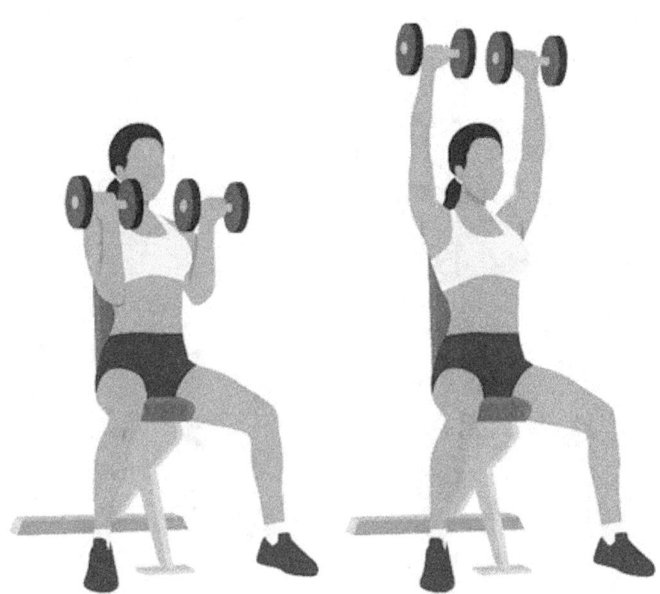

Arnold Press (standing or seated)

- *Muscles Targeted:* Triceps, Shoulders, Neck
- *Instructions:* With elbows bent, hold a dumbbell in each hand with your palms facing your body. Rotate your palms to face forward as you press the dumbbells overhead. Reverse the motion.

Wall Angels

- *Muscles Targeted:* Shoulders, back, neck
- *Instructions:* Using parallel bars or the edge of a sturdy chair, lower your body by bending your elbows, then push back up.

Lower Body/Core Exercises

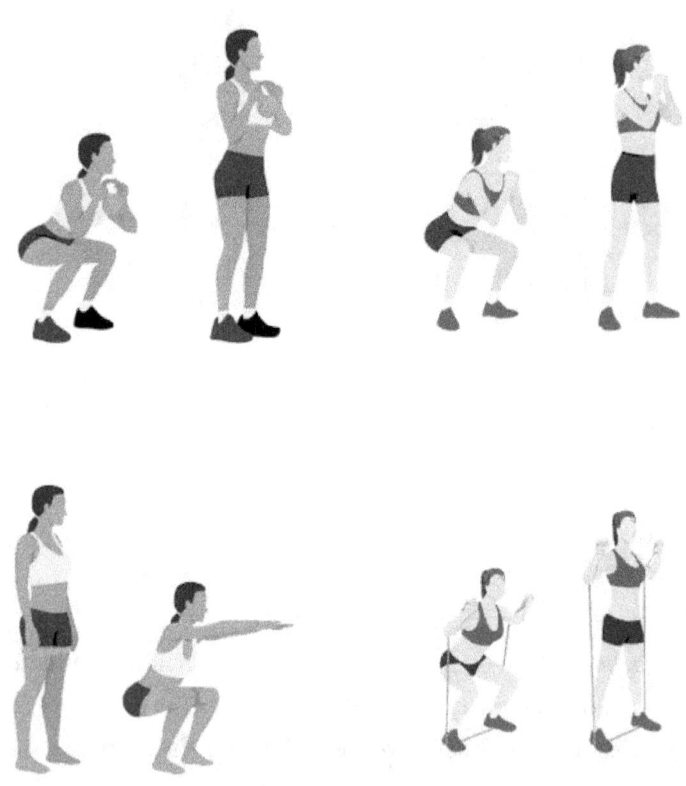

Top left: squat with kettlebell; top right: bodyweight squat; bottom left: squat with resistance band; bottom right: squat with resistance band (tube)

Squats

- *Muscles Targeted:* Quadriceps, hamstrings, glutes
- *Instructions:* Hold a dumbbell or kettlebell in front of your chest. If using a resistance band, either place it around your thighs or stand on it shoulder length apart and hold the handles. You can also do these unassisted using only your bodyweight with your hands at your waist, straightout in front of you, or clasped in front of you. Sit back into a squat as if you're sitting in a chair (or deeper if you can) keeping knees over ankles. Stand back up.
- *Notes: To perform a mini squat* stand with feet shoulder-width apart. Lower your body to approx. 45 degrees ensuring your knees don't go past your toes.

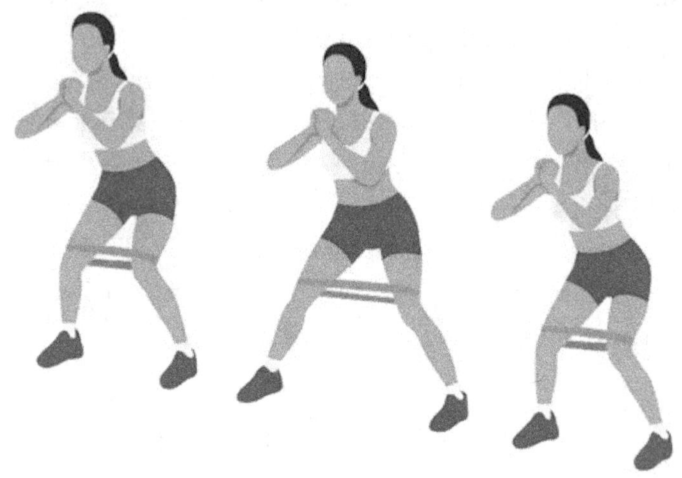

Resistance Band Lateral Walks

- *Muscles Targeted:* Hips, glutes, thighs
- *Instructions:* Place a resistance band around your thighs. Take lateral (to the side) steps, maintaining tension in the bands. Return to the starting position.

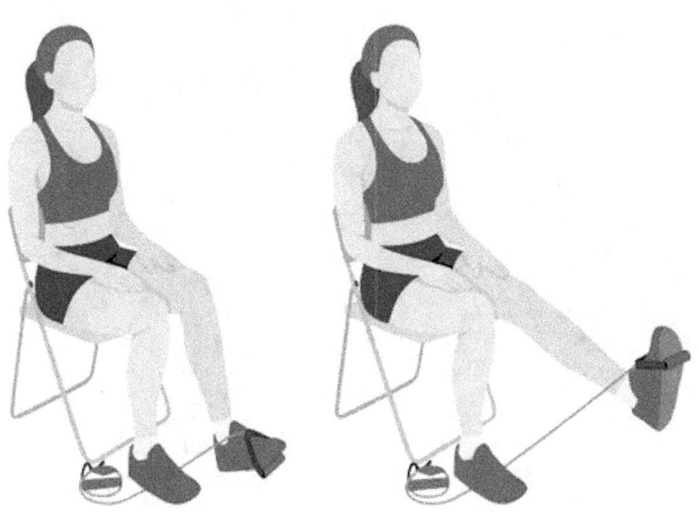

Seated Leg Extensions

- *Muscles Targeted:* Quadriceps
- *Instructions:* Sit on a chair, loop band around one foot or place a band around your ankles. Extend your leg against the resistance. Lower your leg.

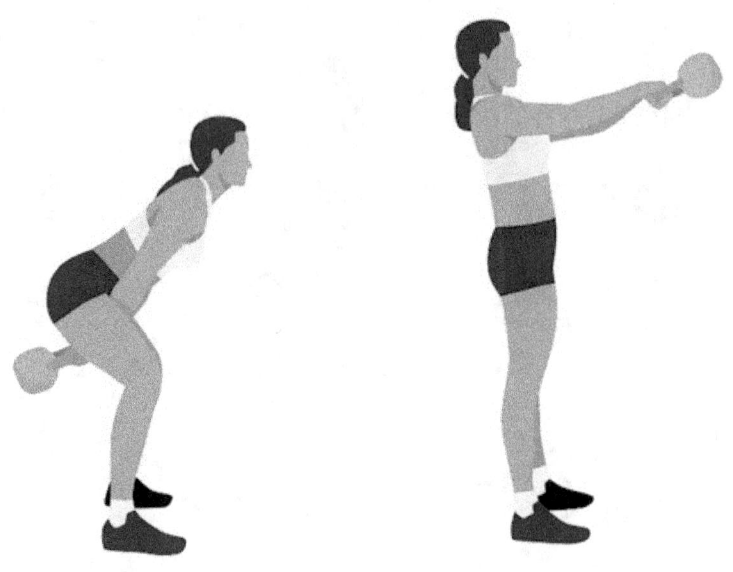

Kettlebell Swing

- *Muscles Targeted:* Hamstrings, Glutes, Core
- *Instructions:* From standing, hinge at your hips, swing the kettlebell between your legs, then thrust your hips forward to swing it to chest height.
- *Notes:* Maintain a neutral spine and use your hips for power.

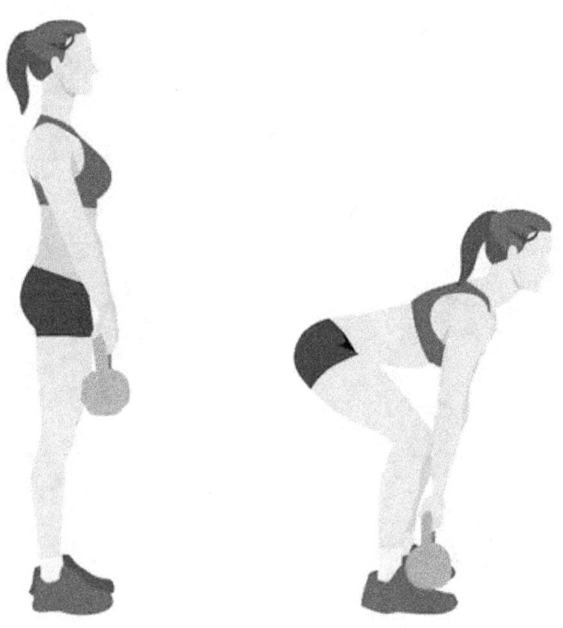

Deadlift

- *Muscles Targeted:* Hamstrings, Glutes, Lower Back
- *Instructions:* Hinge at your hips and keep your back flat. Lower the kettlebell to the ground while keeping it close to your body.
- *Notes:* Maintain a neutral spine and engage your core. Can be done with a dumbbell or resistance bands.

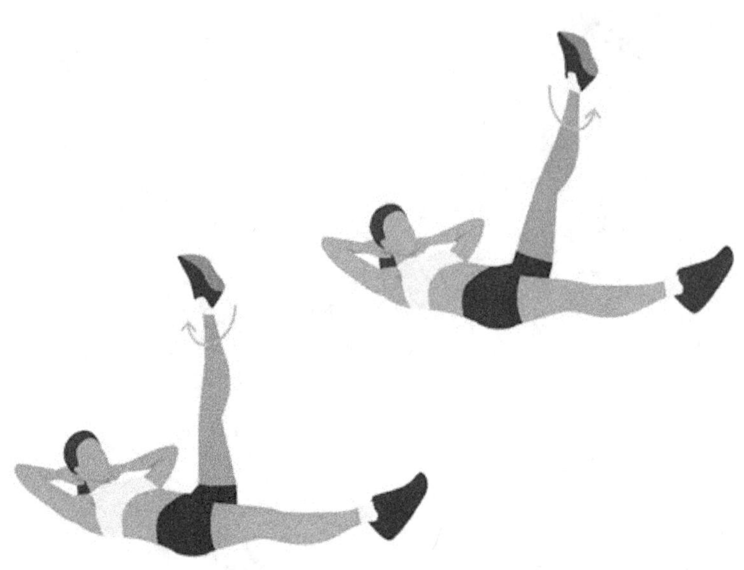

Leg Circles

- *Muscles Targeted:* Core, Hip Flexors
- *Instructions:* Lie on your back, and extend both legs straight or bent at the knee. Lift one leg and draw circles with it. Switch direction.

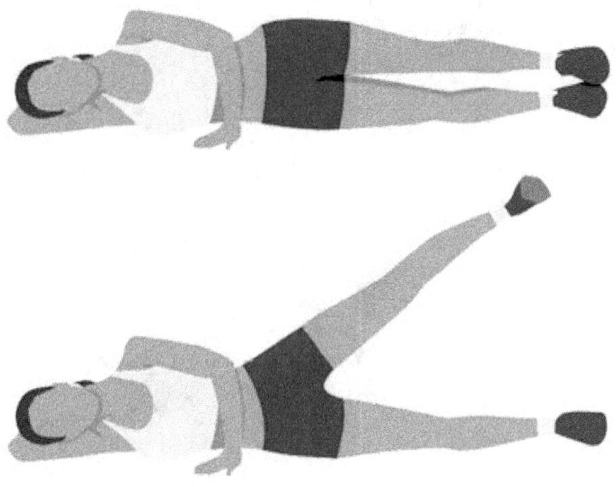

Side-Lying Leg Lifts

- *Muscles Targeted:* Outer Thighs, Abductors
- *Instructions:* Lie on your side, lift and lower the top leg. Switch sides.

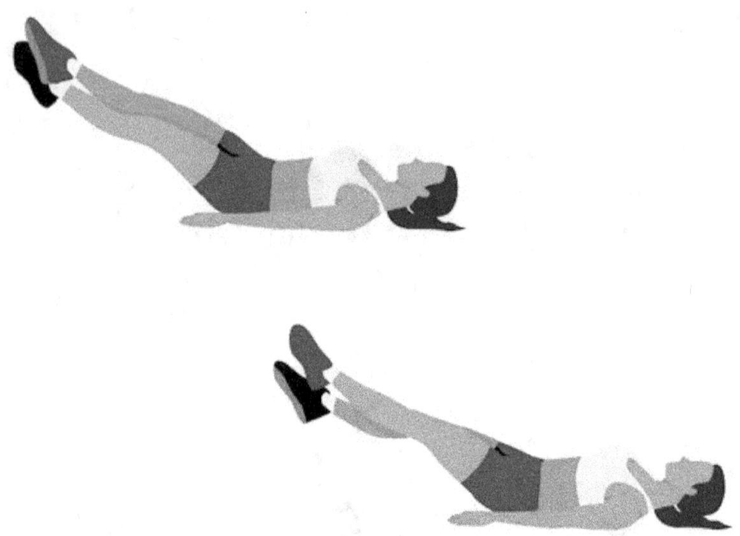

Scissor Kicks

- *Muscles Targeted:* Legs, Lower Abdominals
- *Instructions:* Lie on your back, lift legs, and crisscross them in the air.

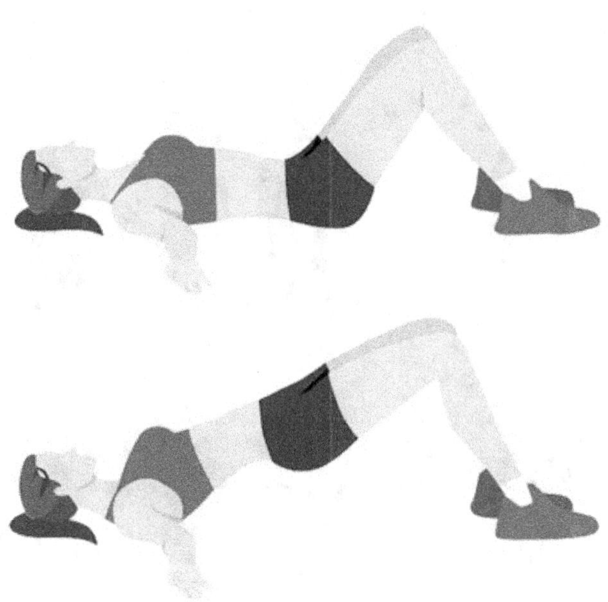

Glute Bridges

- *Muscles Targeted:* Glutes, hamstrings, lower back
- Instructions: Lie on your back with knees bent and feet flat. Lift your hips toward the ceiling, squeezing your glutes. Lower and repeat for 15-20 reps.

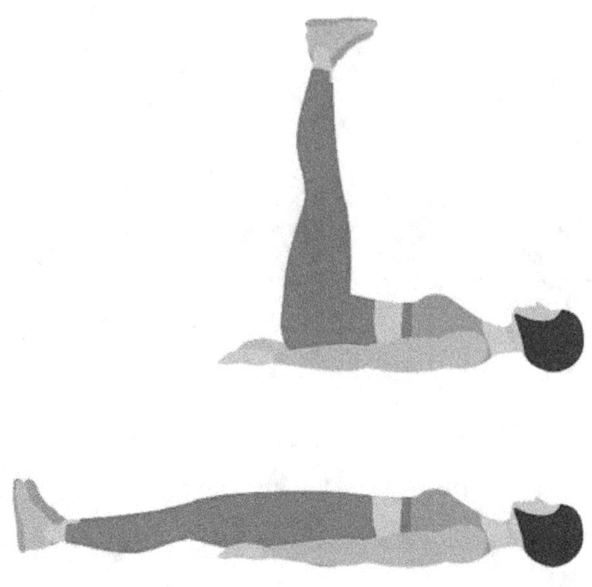

Lying Leg Raises

- *Muscles Targeted:* Lower abs
- *Instructions:* Lie on your back with legs straight. Lift your legs toward the ceiling, then lower them without touching the floor.

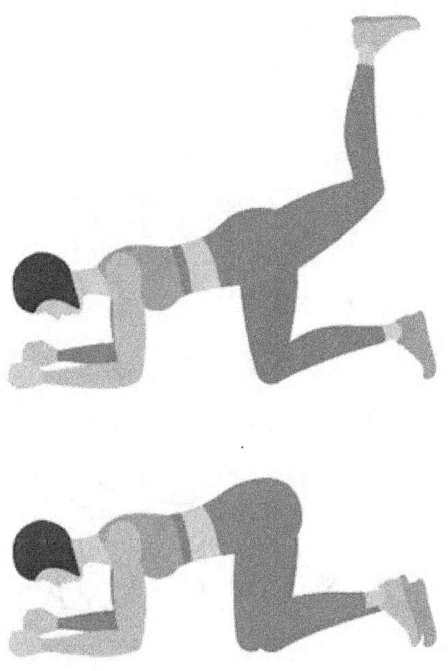

Donkey Kicks

- *Muscles Targeted:* Glutes, hamstrings
- *Instructions:* Start on your hands and knees. Lift one leg toward the ceiling, keeping the knee bent. Lower and repeat, then switch legs.

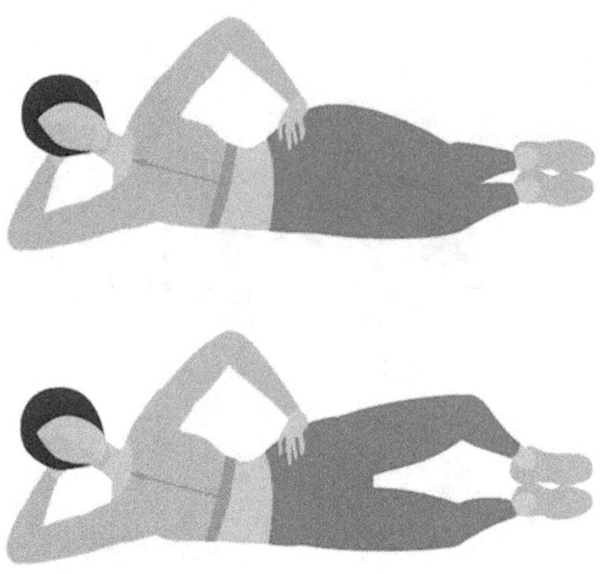

Clamshells

- *Muscles Targeted:* Glutes, hips
- *Instructions:* Lie on your side with knees bent. Keeping your feet together, open and close your knees.

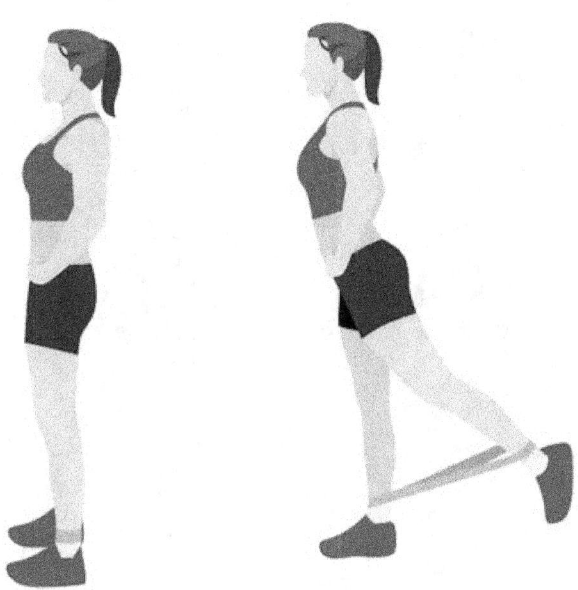

Standing Kickbacks

- *Muscles Targeted:* Glutes, hamstrings
- *Instructions:* Stand with feet hip-width apart with banded ankles. Lift one leg straight back, engaging the glutes. Lower and repeat.

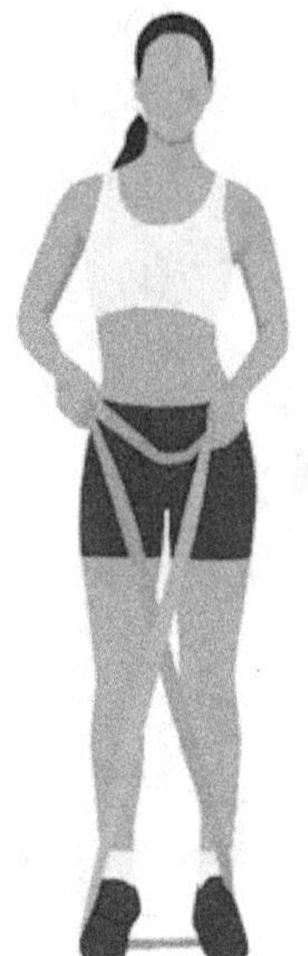 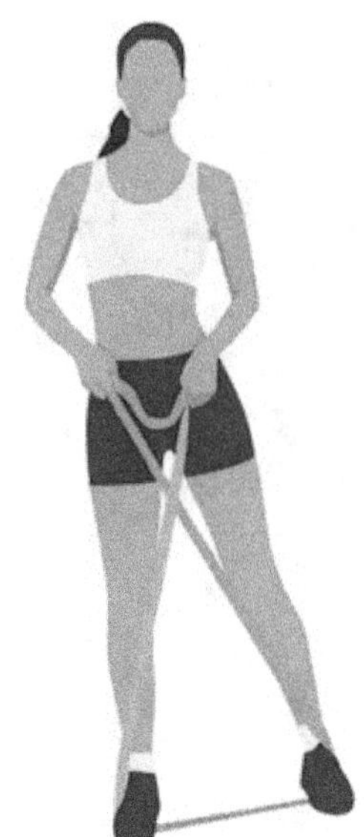

Standing Outer Thigh Raises

- *Muscles Targeted:* Outer thighs, hips
- *Instructions:* Standing with feet shoulder-length apart, place a band under your feet or around your ankles. Lift one leg to the side, then lower maintaining the resistance in the band.

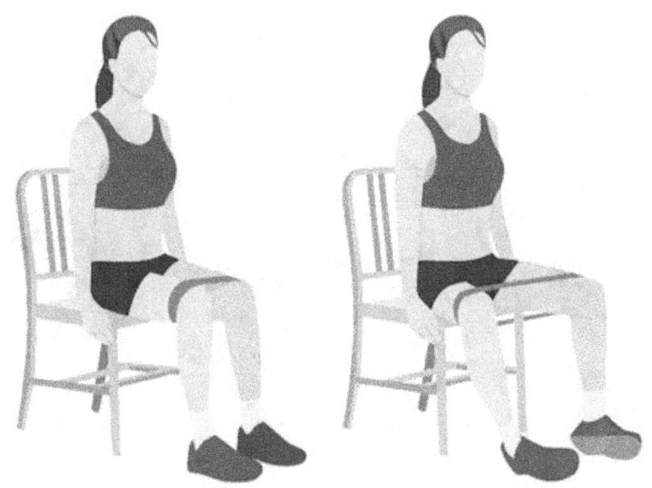

Seated Abductions

- *Muscles Targeted:* Inner thighs
- *Instructions:* Sit in a chair. With a band around your thighs, open and close your legs, engaging your inner thighs.

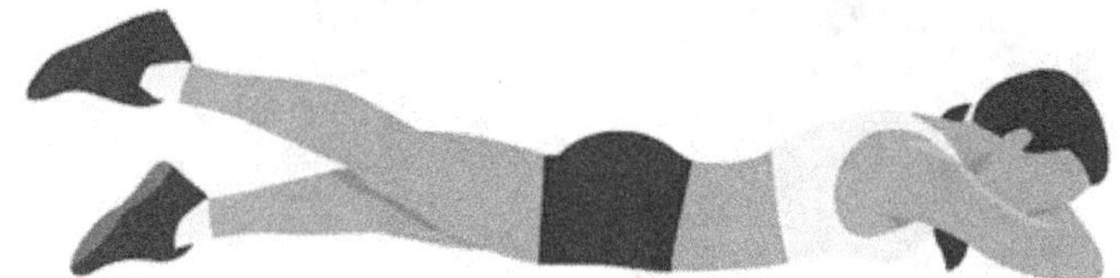

Prone Lying Leg Raises

- *Muscles Targeted:* Glutes, hamstrings
- *Instructions:* Lie on your stomach. Lift one leg off the ground, then lower it.

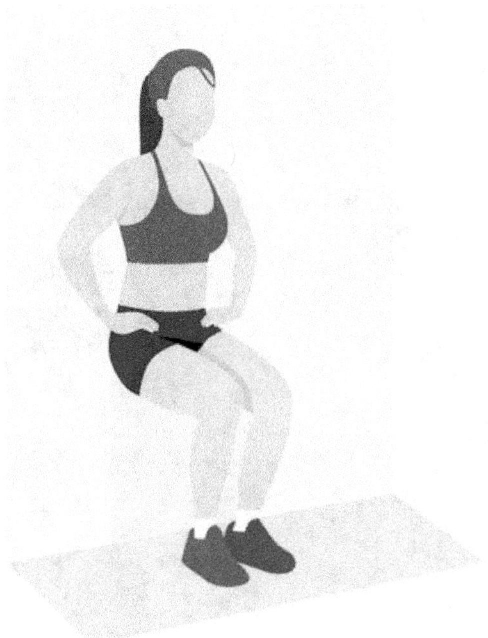

Wall Sit

- *Muscles Targeted:* Quadriceps, hamstrings, glutes
- *Instructions:* Lean against a wall with your feet shoulder-width apart and slide down into a seated position. Keep your back against the wall, thighs parallel to the ground, and knees at a 90-degree angle. Hold the position.

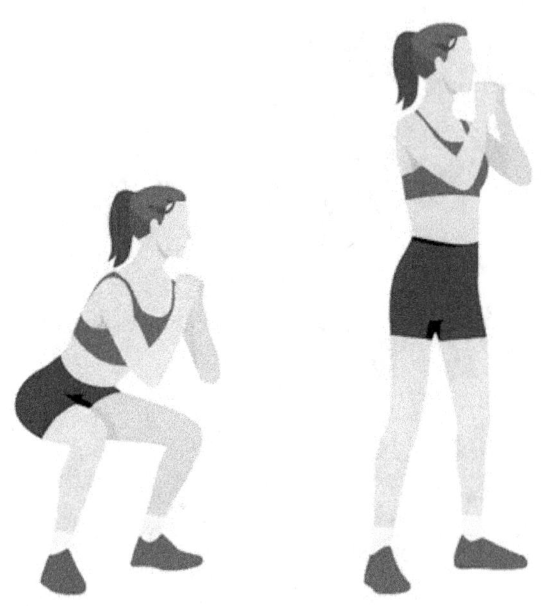

Wall-Assisted Squats with Fitness Ball

- *Muscles Targeted:* Quadriceps, hamstrings, glutes, core
- Instructions: Place a fitness ball between your lower back and the wall. Perform squats by lowering your body, keeping contact with the ball, and pushing through your heels.

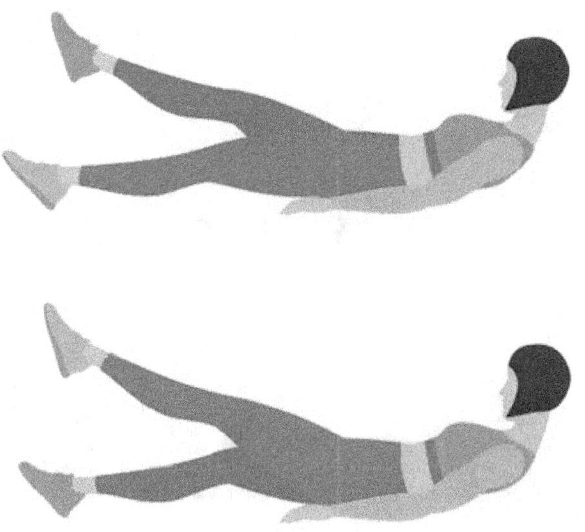

Flutter Kicks

- *Muscles Targeted:* Lower abs, hip flexors
- *Instructions:* Lie on your back, legs straight. Lift your legs a few inches off the ground and flutter them up and down in a controlled motion.

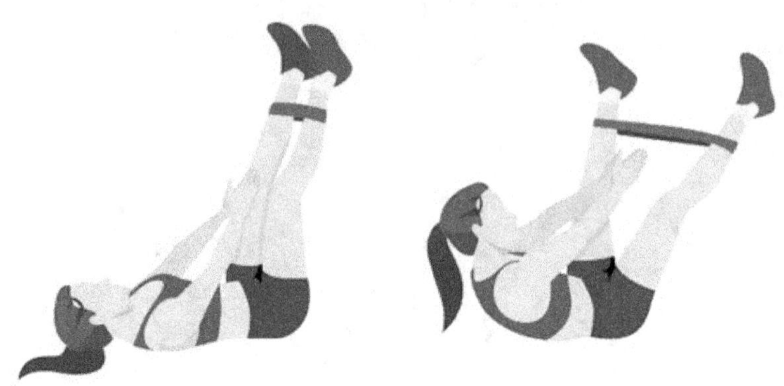

Lying Leg Abduction Crunch

- *Muscles Targeted:* Outer Thighs
- *Instructions:* Lie on your back with a resistance band looped around your ankles or shins. With your legs extended upward, spread your legs while lifting your shoulders to reach for the band with your hands. Lower yourself back to the floor.

Knee Circles

- *Muscles Targeted:* Knee joint mobility
- *Instructions:* Stand with your hands on your knees and make circular motions with your knees, focusing on a smooth range of motion.

Seated Knee Lifts

- *Muscles Targeted:* Quadriceps
- *Instructions:* Sit on the edge of a chair with your back straight. Lift one knee toward your chest and then lower it. Switch legs.

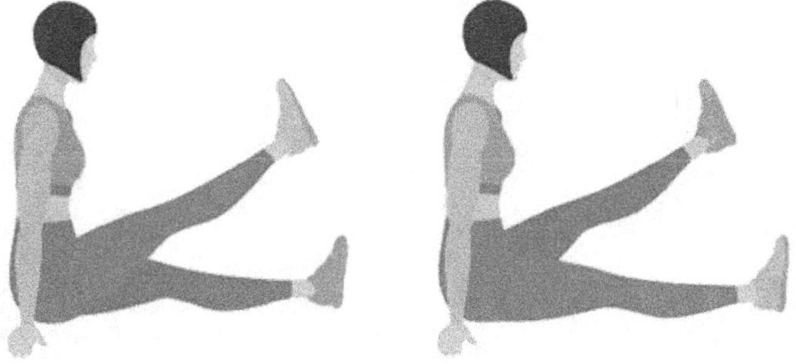

Seated Leg Raises

- *Muscles Targeted:* Quadriceps, hip flexors
- *Instructions:* Sit in a chair or on the floor with your back straight. Lift one leg, extending it straight in front. Lower it back down. Alternate legs.

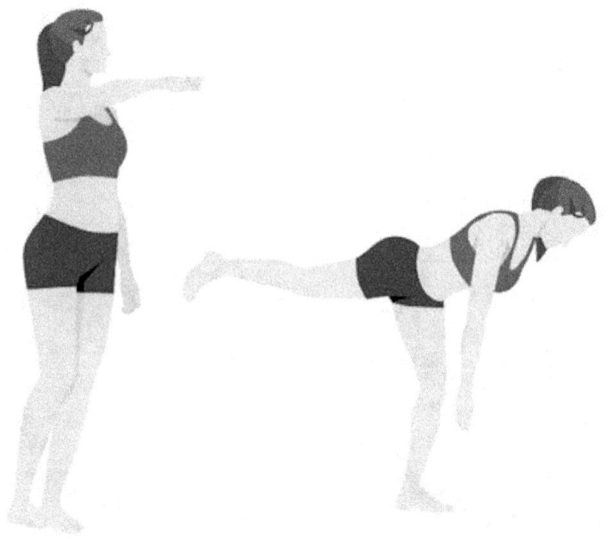

Single Leg Deadlift

- *Muscles Targeted:* Hamstrings, Glutes
- *Instructions:* Stand with your feet flat and your right arm up. Hinge at the hips, lift your right leg to the back, and reach toward the ground. Return to the starting position.

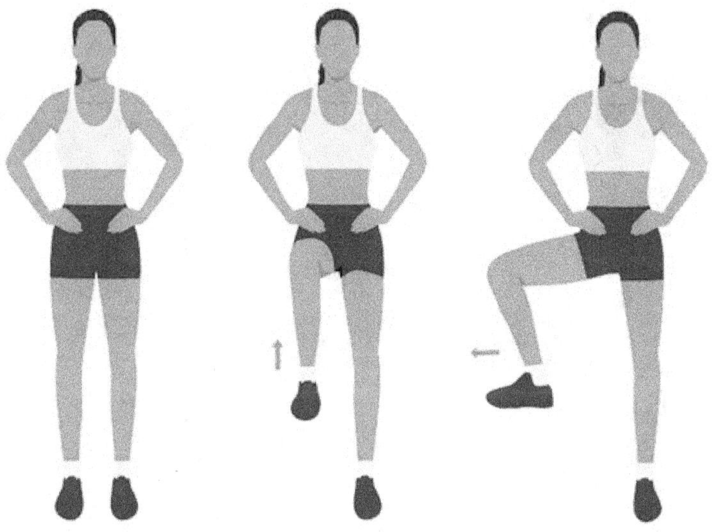

Single Leg Gate Openers

- *Muscles Targeted:* Inner Thighs
- *Instructions:* From standing, lift one knee up and swing it out to the side. Swing it back. Alternate legs.

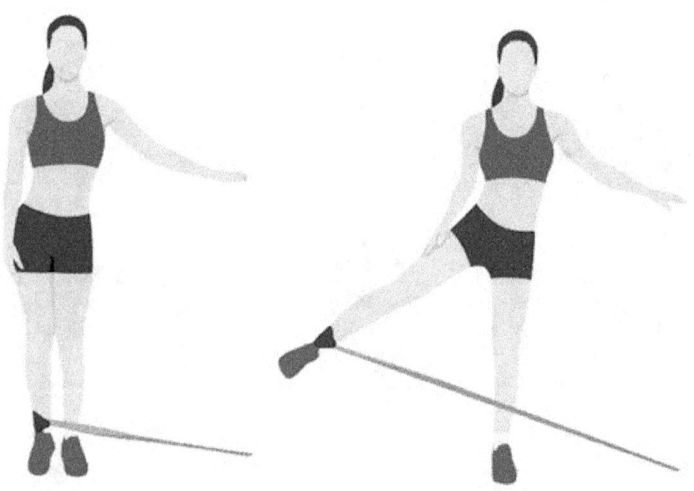

Standing Abduction

- *Muscles Targeted:* Outer Thighs
- *Instructions:* Stand, loop a resistance band around your thighs or ankles, and lift one leg to the side. Return to the starting position. Alternate legs.

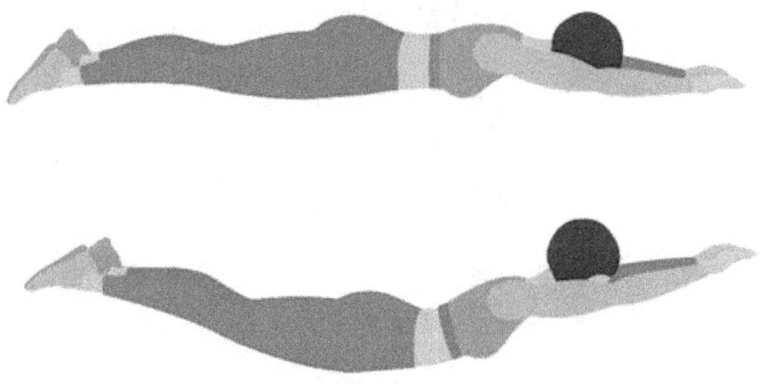

Superman Raises

- *Muscles Worked:* Lower back, rhomboids, traps
- *Instructions:* Lie face down with legs and arms fully extended. Lift

both your legs and arms simultaneously off the ground, squeezing your upper back muscles. Lower to starting.

Cool-down Exercises

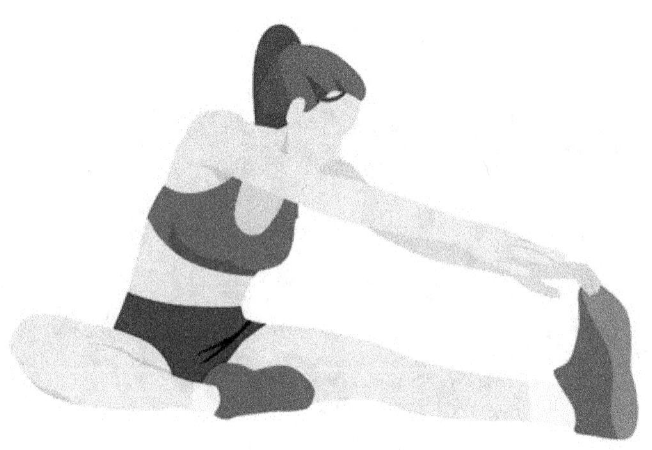

Seated Hamstring Stretch

- *Muscles Targeted:* Hamstrings
- *Instructions:* Sit on the floor, extend one leg, reach towards toes, keeping back straight. Repeat with the other leg.

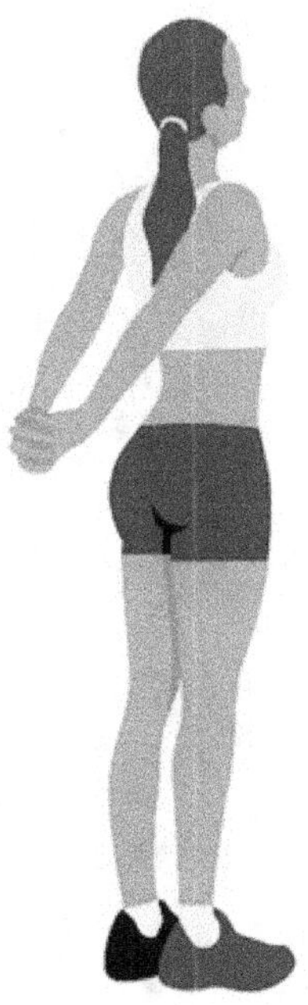

Standing Reverse Shoulder Stretch

- *Muscles Targeted:* Shoulders, upper back, triceps
- *Instructions:* Standing with your back straight, clasp your hands behind your back, and lift your arms towards the ceiling

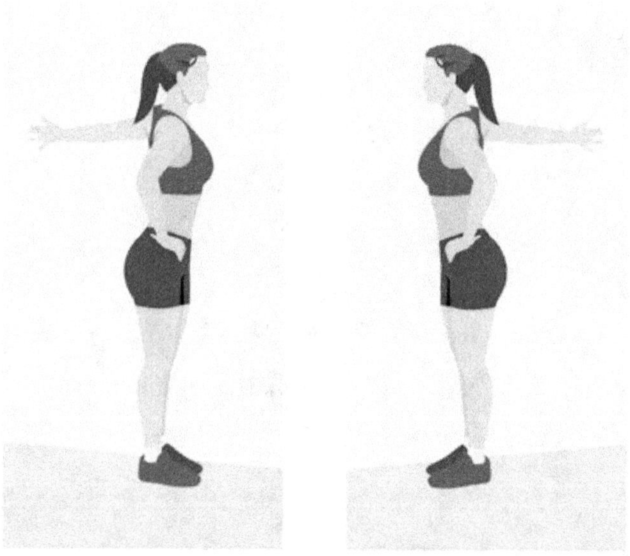

Wall-Assisted Chest Stretch

- *Muscles Targeted:* Chest, front shoulder
- *Instructions:* Stand facing the wall and place your palm flat against the wall. Gently turn your body away from the wall, maintaining contact with your palm, feeling a stretch across your chest and the front of your shoulder. Switch sides.

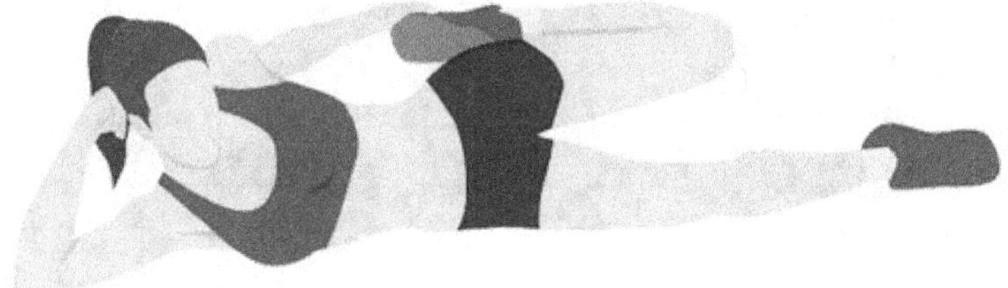

Side-Lying Quad Stretch

- *Muscles Targeted:* Quadriceps
- *Instructions:* Lie on one side, pull your heel toward your glutes, and hold.
- *Notes:* Keep your knees close together.

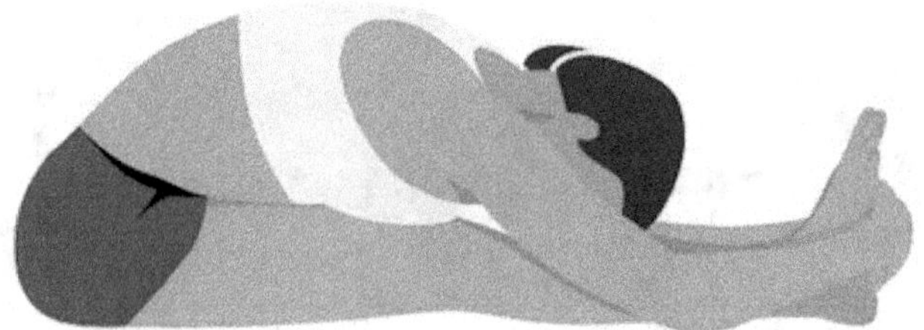

Seated Forward Bend

- *Muscles Targeted:* Hamstrings, Lower Back
- *Instructions:* Sit with both legs extended, lean forward at the hips, reaching toward your toes.
- *Notes:* Keep your back straight and go to a comfortable stretch.

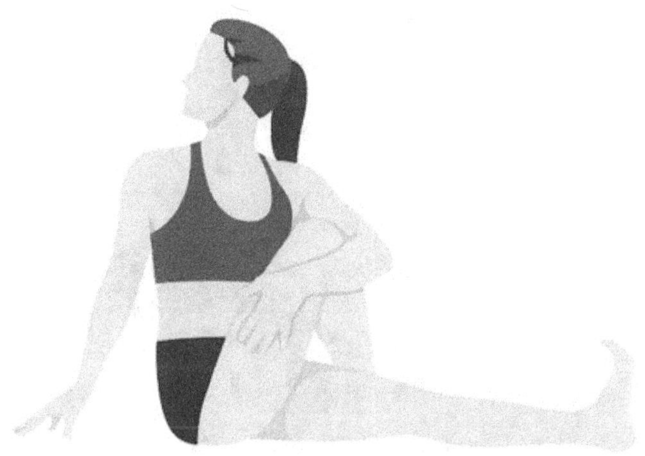

Seated Torso Stretch

- *Muscles Targeted:* Obliques
- *Instructions:* Sit with your legs extended and one leg crossed over the other. Twist your torso to one side and hold.
- *Notes:* Keep your back tall and feel the stretch along your sides.

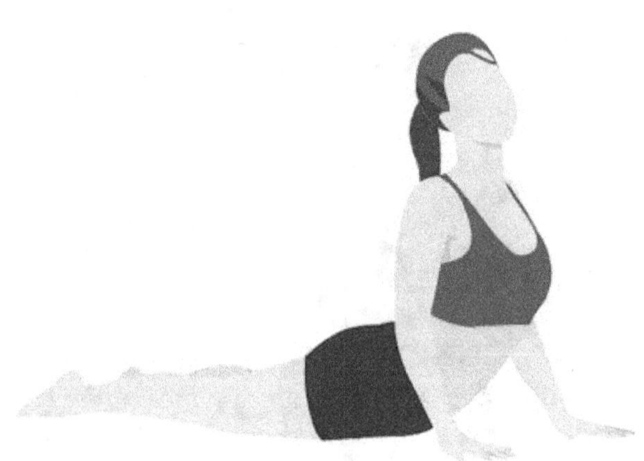

Cobra Pose

- *Muscles Targeted:* Back, Chest
- *Instructions:* Lie on your stomach, push your upper body off the ground, and look upward.
- *Notes:* Lift with your back, not just your hands.

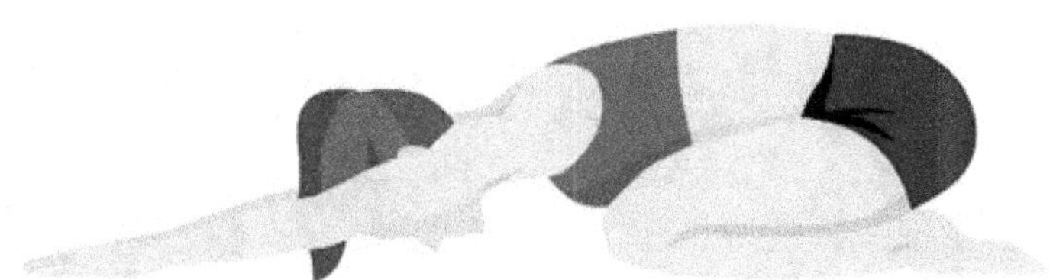

Child's Pose

- *Muscles Targeted:* Back, Shoulders
- *Instructions:* Kneel, sit back on your heels, and reach your arms forward.
- *Notes:* Relax into the stretch, focusing on your breath.

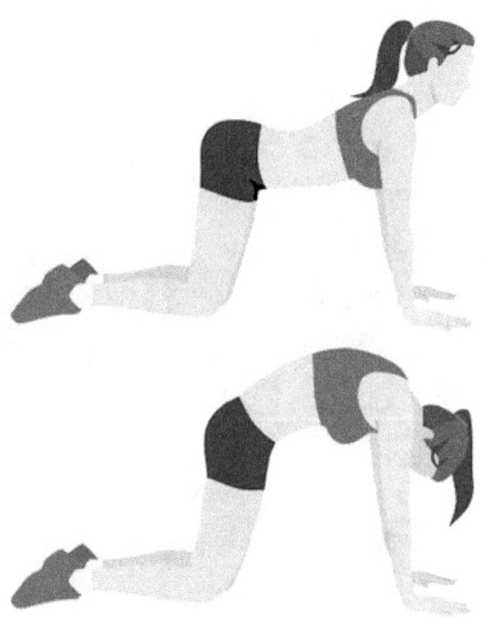

Cat-Cow Stretch

- *Muscles Targeted:* Spine, Abdominals
- *Instructions:* Start on hands and knees. Inhale, arch your back (Cow). Exhale, round your back (Cat).

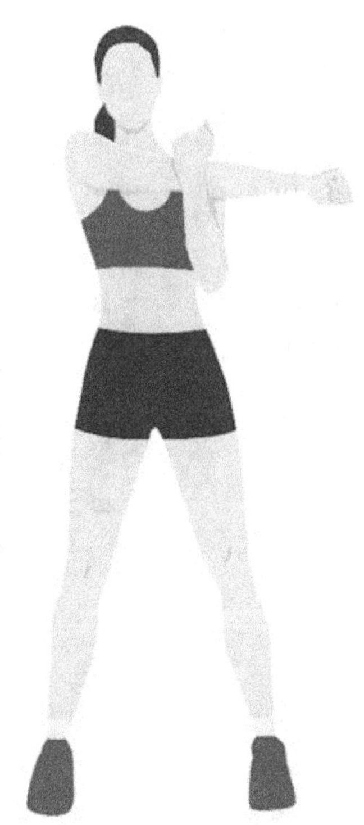

Standing Cross-Body Arm Stretch

- *Muscles Targeted:* Shoulders, Upper Back
- *Instructions:* Stand with your feet shoulder-width apart, extend your right arm straight across your chest at the shoulder and use your left hand to gently pull your right arm closer to your chest until you feel a comfortable stretch. Repeat with the other arm.

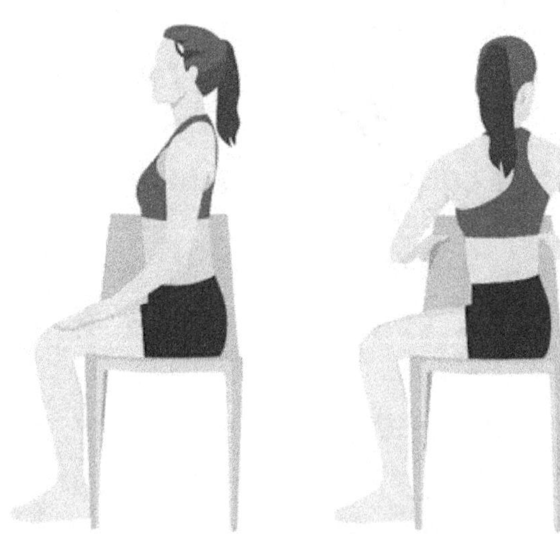

Seated Spine Stretch

- *Muscles Targeted:* Spine, Hamstrings
- *Instructions:* Sit in a chair or on the floor. Twist torso to one side and hold. Repeat on the other side.

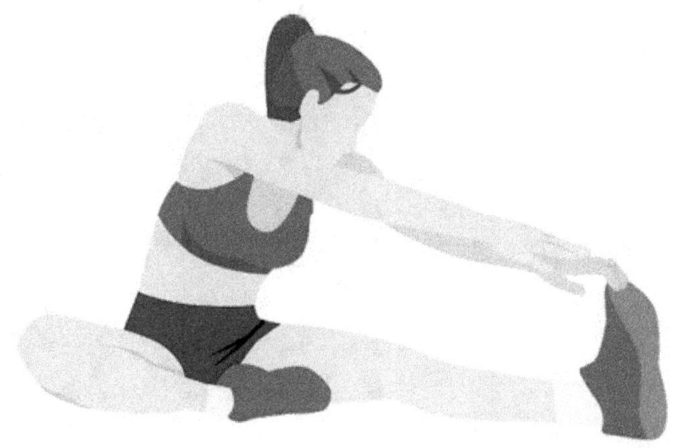

Seated Single-Leg Forward Bend

- *Muscles Targeted:* Hamstrings, Lower Back
- *Instructions:* Sit with one leg extended and one tucked in. Hinge at the hips and reach for your toes on the extended leg. Repeat with the other leg.

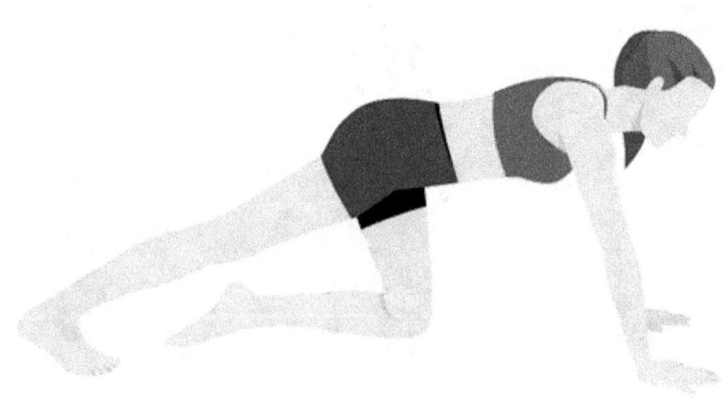

Tabletop Calf Stretch

- *Muscles Targeted:* Calves
- *Instructions:* Get in a tabletop position. Extend one leg backwards with your heel stretched to the ground until you feel a comfortable stretch to the calf. Repeat on other leg.

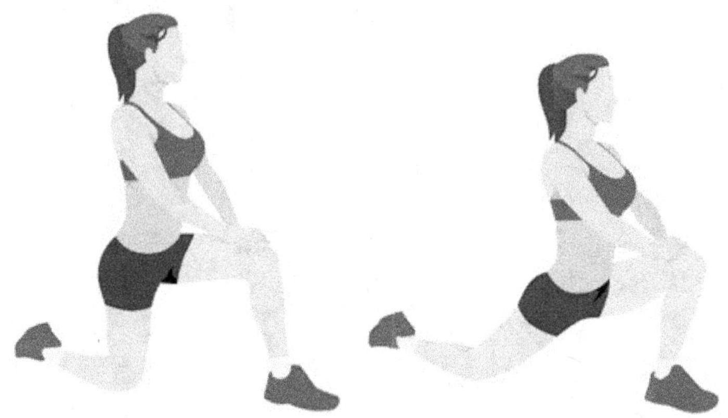

Kneeling Hip Flexor Stretch

- *Muscles Targeted:* Hip flexors, quadriceps
- *Instructions:* Kneeling with one foot forward in a 90-degree angle, shift your weight forward slightly feeling a stretch in the hip of the back leg.

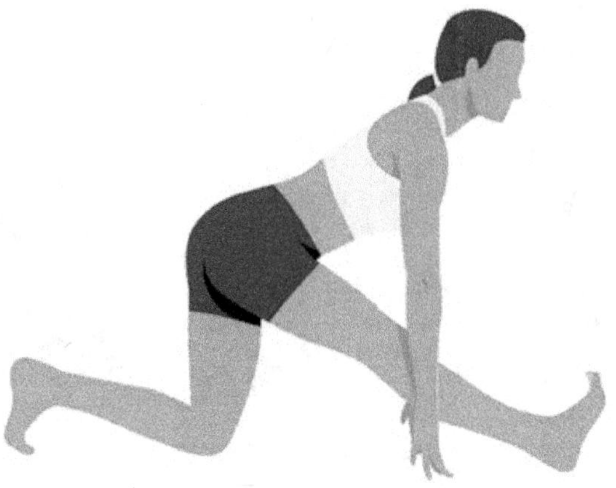

Kneeling Hamstring Stretch

- *Muscles Targeted:* Hamstrings
- *Instructions:* Kneel on one knee with the other foot extended straight in front of you. Hinge at the hips, leaning forward so that your fingertips are on the floor on both sides of your leg until you feel a stretch along the back of the extended leg.

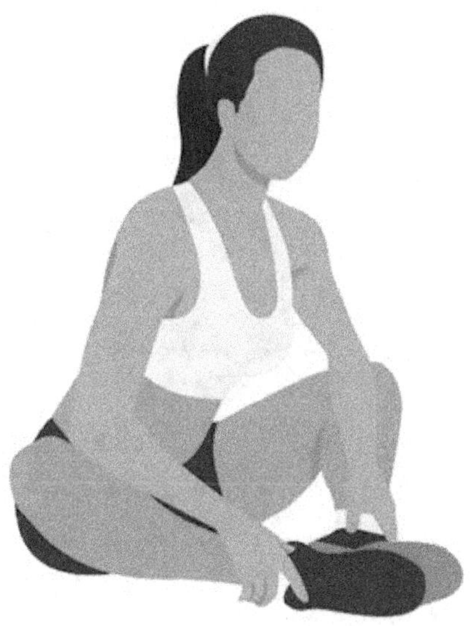

Seated Butterfly

- *Muscles Targeted:* Inner thighs, groin
- *Instructions:* Seated on the floor with your back straight, bring the soles of your feet together allowing your knees to fall to the sides. Hold your feet with your hands and gently press your knees toward the floor until you feel a comfortable stretch along your inner thigh.

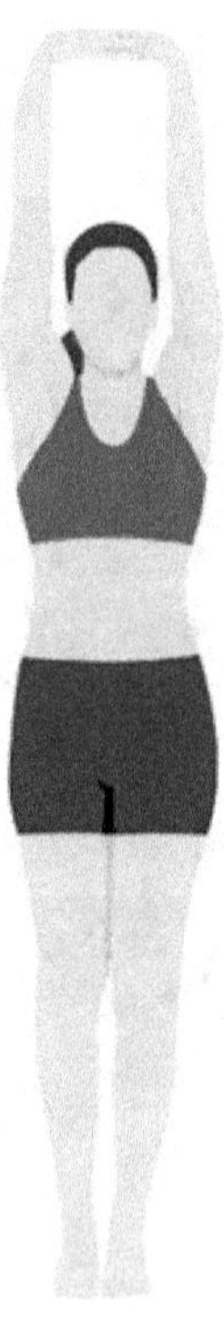

Overhead Stretch

- *Muscles Targeted:* Shoulder, upper back
- *Instructions:* Stand or sit comfortably. Clasp your hands together and extend your arms overhead reaching towards the ceiling.

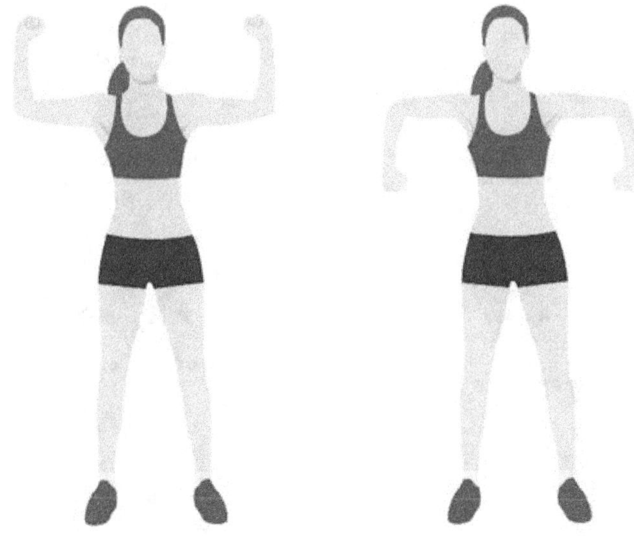

Scarecrow Dynamic Stretch

- *Muscles Targeted:* Shoulder, upper back
- *Instructions:* Standing, bring your arms to the sides at a 90-degree angle. Swivel your arms downward maintaining the 90-degree angle. Repeat.

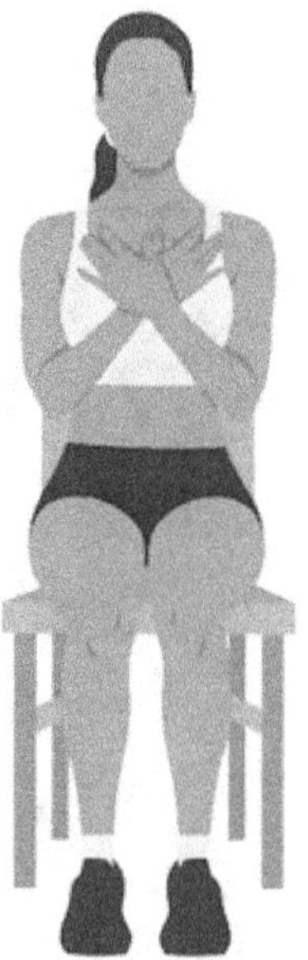 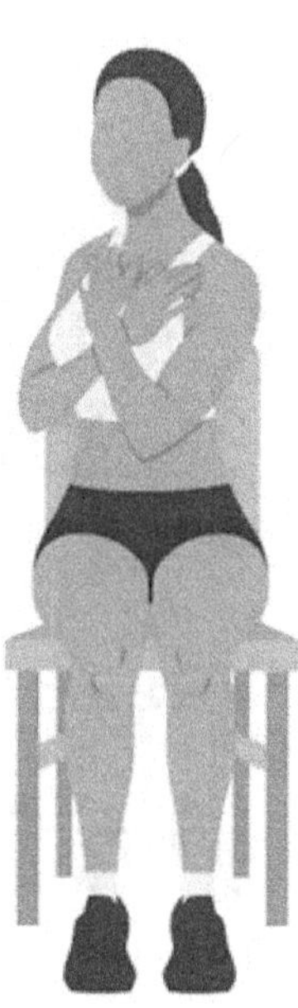

Glute and Lumbar Rotation Stretch

- *Muscles Targeted:* Glutes, Back
- *Instructions:* Seated, cross your wrists at your chest. Twist your torso to one side and hold. Twist to the other side.

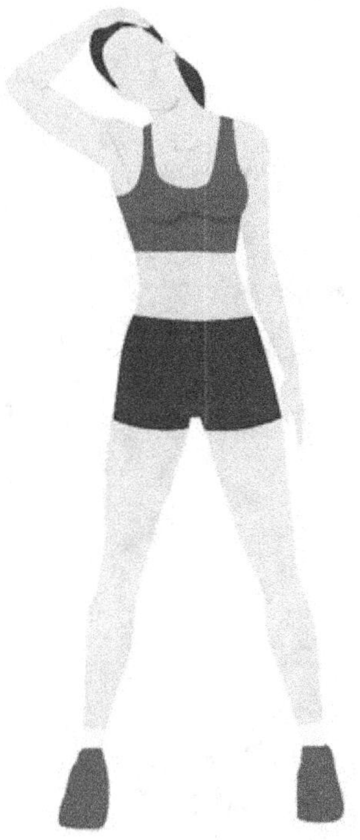

Neck stretch

- *Muscles Targeted:* Neck
- *Instructions:* Sit or stand with a straight spine. Tilt your head to one side, bringing your ear toward your shoulder and drop the other shoulder toward the floor.

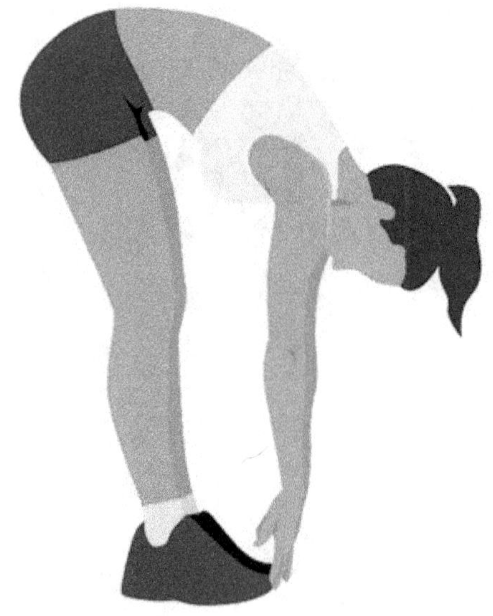

Standing Forward Bend

- *Muscles Targeted:* Hamstrings, lower back
- *Instructions:* Stand with legs extended. Hinge at your hips, reaching toward your toes. Hold.

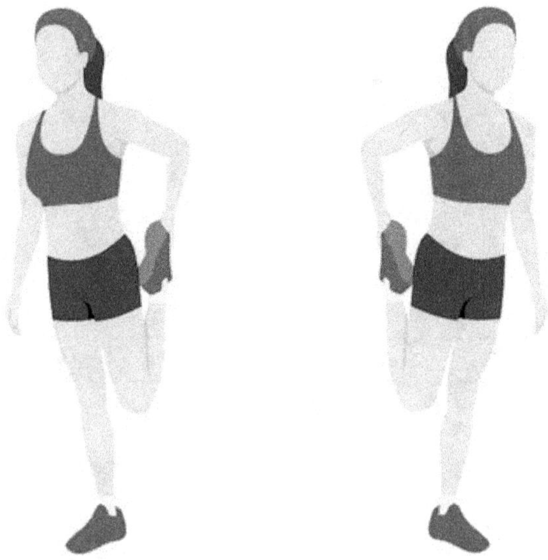

Standing Quad Stretch

- *Muscles Targeted:* Quadriceps
- *Instructions:* Stand on one leg. Bend the other leg, bringing your heel toward your buttocks. Hold, then switch legs.

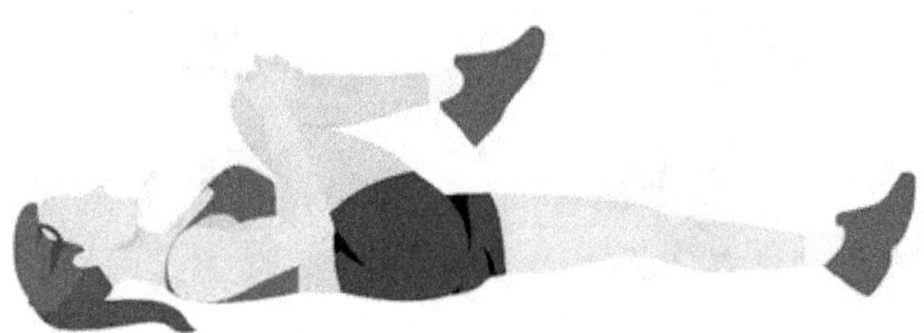

Knee-to-Chest-Stretch

- *Muscles Targeted:* Lower back, hamstrings
- *Instructions:* Lie on your back and bring one knee toward your chest. Hold, then switch legs.

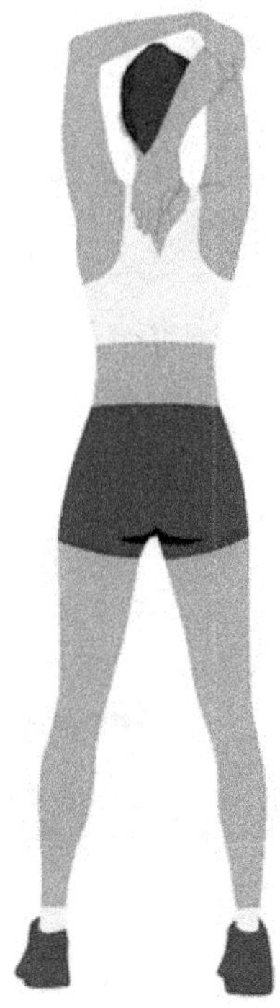

Overhead Tricep Stretch

- *Muscles Targeted:* Triceps
- *Instructions:* Raise one arm overhead, bending the elbow and reaching your hand down your back so that your palm is touching your back. With your other hand, gently grasp your bended elbow and apply gentle pressure, encouraging the stretch in your right tricep. Hold the stretch.

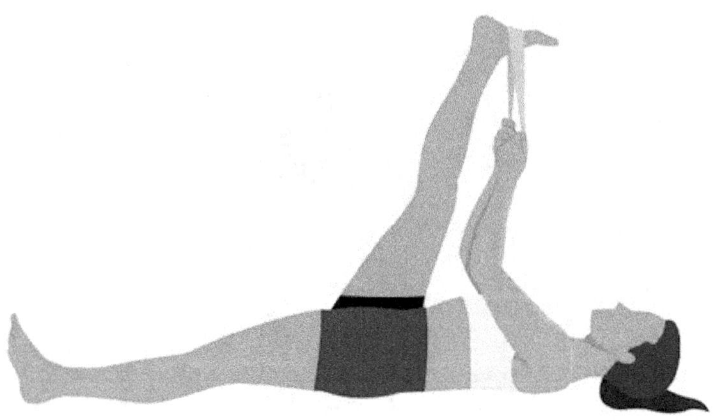

Lying Hamstring Stretch

- *Muscles Targeted:* Hamstrings
- *Instructions:* Lie on your back, lift one leg and gently pull it toward your face with your hands, a resistance band, or a stretch strap. You can even use a towel or a t-shirt.

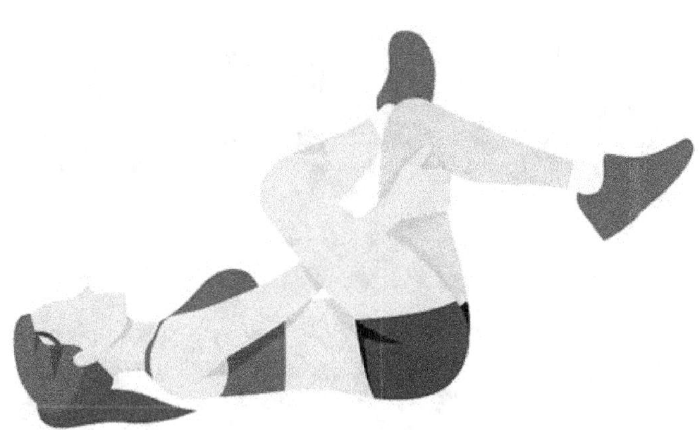

Lying Glute Stretch

- *Muscles Targeted:* Glutes
- *Instructions:* Lie on your back, cross one ankle over the opposite knee, and gently pull the knee towards your chest until you feel a comfortable stretch.

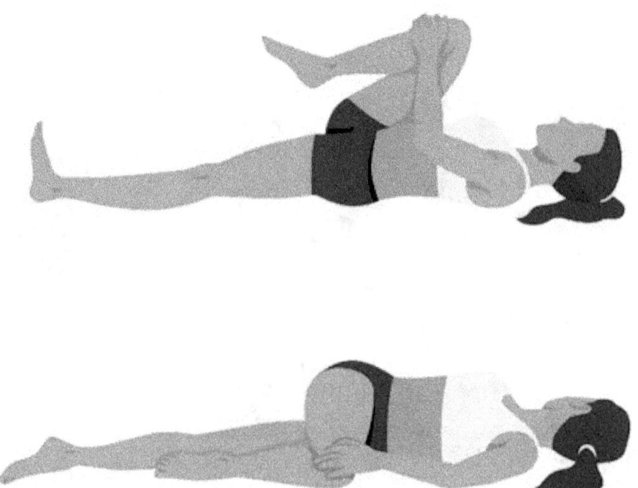

Knee-to-Chest-to-Spine Stretch

- *Muscles Targeted:* Glutes
- *Instructions: Instructions:* Lie on your back and bring one knee toward your chest. Hold. Swivel the lifted knee and lay it over the other leg to touch the ground. Hold.

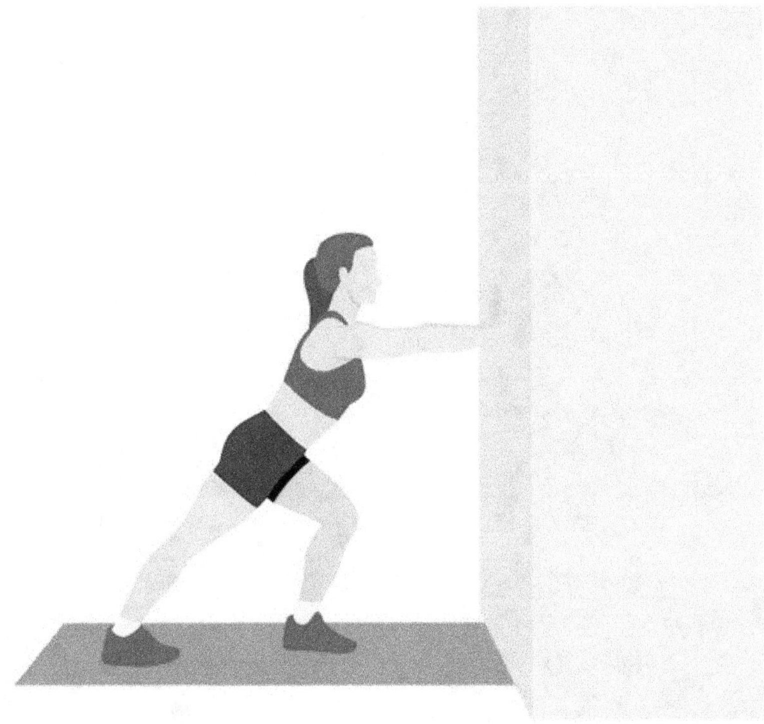

Standing Calf Stretch

- *Muscles Targeted:* Calves
- *Instructions:* Stand near a wall or any stable vertical surface. Rest your hands on the wall at shoulder height. Keeping a slight bend in one knee, step back with the other foot keeping the leg straight and your heel to the floor. Feel a comfortable stretch and hold.

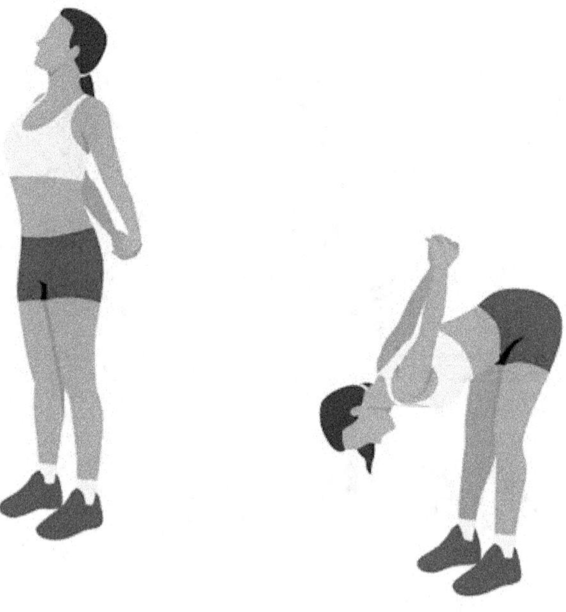

Clasped Arm Extension with Forward Bend

- *Muscles Targeted:* Hamstrings, lower back, shoulders, biceps
- *Instructions:* Stand with feet shoulder length apart. Clasp your hands behind your back keeping them close to your body. Slowly lift your clasped hands towards your upper back and hinge at the waist until in a forward bend

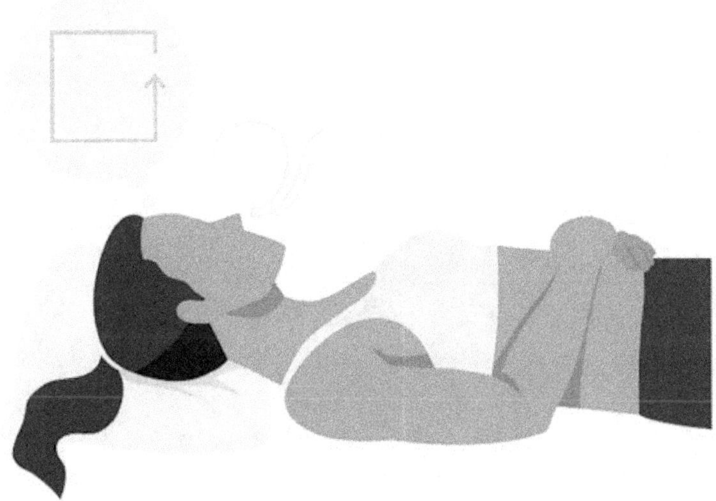

Box Breathing

Muscles targeted: NA (relaxation is the target)

Instructions: inhale for 4 seconds, hold for 4 seconds, exhale for 4 seconds

8

Routines: 15-Minute Knee-Friendly Home Workouts

You made it! Whether you're a beginner or someone easing back into working out, these 15-minute workouts will help you build strength, improve flexibility, and boost overall well-being, all within the comfort of your home. To keep your joints happy (especially those knees), each workout is accompanied by a warm-up and cool-down which may bring the total session to 20 minutes. Depending on how many days you have decided to work out, I encourage you to do 1-2 lower body/core workouts, 1-2 upper body/core workouts, and 1 full body workout per week. I also recommend adding at least one day of cardio to your routine. Get ready to transform your approach to fitness, one short and sweet workout at a time!

How to use this guide

In Chapter 6, you decided what days of the week you are going to work out. Based on that schedule, you will choose a workout that corresponds to the body area and the workout method you've chosen for the day.

For example, if you've decided to do strength training for the upper body today, you will choose a workout from the upper body section, and a cool-down from the cool-down section. Here's a sample workout selection based on the sample week shown in Chapter 6.

Monday (lower body/core): Kettlebell Kickstart

Tuesday (upper body/core): Dumbbell Dynamo

Wednesday (lower body/core): Bodyweight Blast

Thursday (upper body/core): Arm Band-Aid

Friday: rest day

Saturday (full body/core): Pilates Flexi-Flow

Sunday (cardio): 30-minute treadmill walk

Workouts/Routines

Full Body

Workout 1: Dynamic Body Boost

Equipment Needed: dumbbells, resistance bands, mat

Warm-Up:

- Jumping jacks: 1 minute
- Arm circles: 1 minute each direction
- Forward leg swings: 1 minute each leg

Circuit:

- Squats with dumbbell: 12-15 reps
- Bent-over rows with dumbbells: 12-15 reps
- Lateral walks with bands: 10-12 steps each side

- Elbow plank with leg lifts: 10-12 lifts each leg
- Bicep curls with dumbbells: 12-15 reps
- Seated leg extensions with bands: 12-15 reps each leg
- Repeat circuit 1-2x

Cool-Down:

- Seated Hamstring Stretch: 30 second hold each side
- Standing reverse shoulder stretch: 30 second hold each side
- Wall-assisted chest stretch: 30 second hold each side
- Seated single-leg forward bend: 30 second hold each side

Workout 2: Kettlebell Core Blast

Equipment Needed: kettlebell, mat, knee pads (optional)

Warm-Up:

- High knees: 1 minute
- Fingertip-to-toe touches: 1 minute
- Ankle circles: 30 seconds per ankle
- Arm swings: 30 seconds

Circuit:

- Goblet squat to overhead press: 12-15 reps
- Kettlebell swings: 12-15 reps
- Bent-over one-arm row: 10-12 reps each arm
- Push-ups: 12-15 reps
- Deadlift: 12-15 reps
- Repeat circuit 1-2x

Cool-Down:

- Side-lying quad stretch: 30 second hold each side
- Seated forward bend: 30 second hold
- Seated torso stretch: 30 second hold
- Cobra pose: 30 second hold
- Child's pose: 30 second hold

Workout 3: Pilates Flexi-Flow
Equipment Needed: mat, knee pads (optional)

Warm-Up:

- Cat-cow stretch: 1 minute
- Standing cross-body arm stretch: 30 second hold each arm
- Forward leg swings: 1 minute

Circuit:

- Leg circles: 12 reps
- Side-lying leg lifts: 15 reps each side
- Pilates hundred: 1 minute
- Bird-dogs: 12 reps each side
- Scissor kicks: 1 minute
- Seated spine stretch: 12 reps
- Repeat circuit 1-2x

Cool-Down:

- Seated single-leg forward bend: 30 second hold each side

- Tabletop calf stretch: 30 second hold each leg
- Child's pose: 30 second hold
- Box breathing and relaxation: 1-2 minutes

Workout 4: Good Morning Stretch

Equipment Needed: mat, knee pads (optional)

Warm-Up:

- March in place: 1 minute
- Lateral leg swings: 30 seconds each leg
- Hip circles: 30 seconds each direction
- Calf raises: 1 minute
- Ankle circles: 30 seconds each ankle

Circuit:

- Glute and lumbar rotation stretch: 30 seconds each side
- Seated spine stretch: 30 seconds each side
- Neck stretch: 30 seconds each side
- Kneeling hip flexor stretch: 30 seconds each leg
- Kneeling hamstring stretch: 30 seconds each leg
- Standing reverse shoulder stretch: 30 seconds
- Overhead stretch: 30 seconds
- Scarecrow dynamic stretch: 30 seconds
- Seated butterfly: 30 seconds
- Cat-cow stretch: 1 minute

Cool-Down:

- Box breathing and relaxation: 1-2 minutes

Lower Body/Core

Workout 5: Kettlebell Kickstart
Equipment Needed: Kettlebell, mat

Warm-Up:

- Jab-cross: 1 minute
- March in place: 1 minute
- Seated leg extensions: 30 seconds each leg
- Seated leg raises: 30 seconds each leg

Circuit:

- Kettlebell swings: 12-15 reps
- Deadlift: 12-15 reps
- Wood chops: 10-12 reps each side
- Russian twists: 12-15 reps
- Side plank: 1 minute each side
- Repeat circuit 1-2x

Cool-Down:

- Seated or standing forward bend: 30 second hold
- Ankle circles: 30 seconds each ankle
- Standing quad stretch: 30 second hold each leg
- Tabletop calf stretch: 30 second hold each leg

Workout 6: Bodyweight Blast
Equipment Needed: cardio machine (optional), mat, knee pads

(optional)

Warm-Up:

- Cardio (walk outside, treadmill, elliptical, bike, etc.): 5 minutes

Circuit:

- Single leg deadlifts: 12-15 reps each side
- Glute bridges: 15-20 reps
- Forearm plank: 1 minute
- Lying leg raises: 15-20 reps
- Donkey kicks: 15-20 reps alternating
- Clamshells: 12-15 reps each side
- Repeat circuit 1-2x

Cool-Down:

- Seated torso stretch: 30 second hold each side
- Knee-to-chest stretch: 30 second hold each side
- Lying glute stretch: 30 second hold each side

Workout 7: Resistance Band Revitalize

Equipment Needed: resistance bands, mat, jump rope (optional)

Warm-Up:

- Arm circles: 30 seconds each direction
- Lateral leg swings: 30 second each leg
- Hip circles: 30 seconds each direction
- Seated spine stretch: 30 seconds each side

- Jumping rope (real or imaginary): 1 minute

Circuit:

- Lateral walks with bands: 10-12 steps each direction
- Standing kickbacks: 12-15 reps each leg
- Outer thigh raises: 12-15 reps each leg
- Seated abductions: 15-20 reps
- Bicycle crunches: 15-20 reps
- Repeat circuit 1-2x

Cool-Down:

- Knee-to-chest-to-spine stretch: hold Knee-to-chest 30 seconds, hold spine 30 seconds, repeat on other side
- Seated or standing forward bend: 30 second hold
- Standing quad stretch: 30 second hold each side

Workout 8: PowerCore

Equipment Needed: cardio machine (optional), resistance bands, mat, knee pads

(optional)

Warm-Up:

- Cardio (walk outside, treadmill, elliptical, bike, etc.): 5 minutes

Circuit:

- Leg circles: 12-15 reps each leg
- Crunches: 15-20 reps

- Lying leg abduction crunch: 12-15 reps
- Prone lying leg raises: 12-15 each side
- Clamshells: 12-15 each side
- Repeat circuit 1-2x

Cool-Down:

- Kneeling hamstring stretch: 30 second hold each side
- Lying glute stretch: 30 second hold each side
- Cobra pose: 30 second hold
- Child's pose: 30 second hold
- Box breathing and relaxation: 1-2 minutes

Workout 9: Pilates Wonder

Equipment Needed: resistance bands, fitness/stability ball, mat, knee pads (optional)

Warm-Up:

- Butt kicks: 1 minute
- Fingertip-to-toe touches: 1 minute
- hip circles: 30 seconds each direction
- Calf raises: 30 seconds

Circuit:

- Wall sit: 1 minute
- Wall-assisted squats with fitness ball: 12-15 reps
- Single leg gate openers: 12-15 reps each side
- Standing abduction: 12-15 reps each side
- Leg up the wall crunch: 15-20 reps

- Flutter kicks: 12-15 reps
- Repeat circuit 1-2x

Cool-Down:

- Lying hamstring stretch: 30 second hold each side
- Side-lying quad stretch: 30 second hold each side
- Cobra pose: 30 second hold
- Child's pose: 30 second hold
- Box breathing and relaxation: 1-2 minutes

Workout 10: Joint Juice

Equipment Needed: resistance bands, mat

Warm-Up:

- Arm swings: 30 seconds each direction
- Fingertip-to-toe touches: 1 minute
- Lateral leg swings: 30 seconds each side

Circuit:

- Lateral walks with bands: 10-12 steps each side
- Knee circles: 30 seconds each knee
- Seated leg extensions with bands: 12-15 reps each leg
- Mini squats: 1 minute
- Seated knee lifts: 1 minute each knee
- Seated leg raises: 1 minute each leg
- Repeat circuit 1-2x

Cool-Down:

- Standing calf stretch: 30 seconds each leg
- Glute and lumbar rotation stretch: 1 minute
- Knee-to-chest stretch: 30 second hold each side

Upper Body/Core

Workout 11: Dumbbell Dynamo
Equipment Needed: dumbbells

Warm-Up:

- Jumping jacks: 1 minute
- Plank on knees and forearm: 1 minute
- Arm swings: 1 minute

Circuit:

- Overhead press: 12-15 reps
- Bent-over rows: 12-15 reps
- Lateral side shoulder raises: 12-15 reps
- Front arm raises: 12-15 reps
- Hammer grip curls: 12-15 reps
- Tricep extensions: 12-15 reps
- Repeat circuit 1-2x

Cool-Down:

- Standing cross-body arm stretch: 30 second hold each arm
- Overhead tricep stretch: 30 second hold each arm
- Neck stretch: 30 second hold each side

- Clasped arm extension with forward bend: 30 second hold each position
- Standing forward bend: 30 second hold

Workout 12: Arm Band-Aid

Equipment Needed: resistance band and/or Pilates bar, mat, jump rope (optional)

Warm-Up:

- Plank: 1 minute
- Cat-cow stretch: 30 seconds
- Jumping rope: 1 minute
- Step-ups: 1 minute

Circuit:

- Reverse flys: 12-15 reps
- Standing Arnold press: 12-15 reps
- Lateral arm raises: 12-15 reps
- Front arm raises: 12-15 reps
- Tricep dips: 12-15 reps
- Repeat circuit 2x

Cool-Down:

- Standing cross-body arm stretch: 30 second hold each arm
- Overhead tricep stretch: 30 second hold each arm
- Neck stretch: 30 second hold each side
- Overhead stretch: 30 second hold

- Standing forward bend: 30 second hold

Workout 13: Bodyweight Bliss

Equipment Needed: mat, cardio machine (optional), knee pads (optional)

Warm-Up:

- Cardio (walk outside, treadmill, elliptical, bike, etc.): 5 minutes

Circuit:

- Wall angels: 12-15 reps
- Push-ups: 12-15 reps
- Plank: 1 minute
- Superman raises: 12-15 reps
- Pilates swimming: 12-15 reps
- Repeat circuit 1-2x

Cool-Down:

- Clasped arm extension with forward bend: 30 second hold each position
- Standing cross-body arm stretch: 30 second hold each arm
- Cobra pose: 30 second hold
- Child's pose: 30 second hold

9

Conclusion

As we reach the conclusion of "Quick Home Workouts for Women with Bad Knees," it's not just the end of a book but the beginning of a transformative fitness journey. These 15-minute knee-friendly workouts have not only prioritized your joint health but also empowered you to enhance stability, facilitate weight loss, build strength, and boost your energy levels. Through tailored exercises that consider the unique needs of women with knee concerns, you've discovered a sustainable approach to fitness that accommodates different fitness levels and lifestyles.

Remember, it's not about the duration of your workout but the consistency and adaptability it offers. These short and effective sessions have become a catalyst for a positive lifestyle change, proving that investing in your health doesn't require hours of strenuous exercise. By incorporating these quick home workouts into your routine, you've laid the foundation for improved well-being and vitality. So, continue to enjoy the journey, celebrate your progress, and relish the empowerment that comes with taking charge of your fitness, one knee-friendly workout at a time.

If you found this book helpful, I'd be very appreciative if you left a favorable review for the book on Amazon!

References

Baker P, Reading I, Cooper C, Coggon D. Knee disorders in the general population and their relation to occupation. *Occup Environ Med.* 2003;60(10):794-797.

Bunt, C. W., Jonas, C. E., & Chang, J. G. (2018, November 1). *Knee pain in adults and Adolescents: the initial evaluation.* AAFP. https://www.aafp.org/pubs/afp/issues/2018/1101/p576.html#afp20181101p576-b1
   Weak in the knees? (2000, February 20). WebMD. https://www.webmd.com/pain-management/knee-pain/features/weak-in-knees

Burian, C. (2022, January 28). *Doshas: what are they and how can they transform your health?* Kerala Ayurveda USA. https://www.keralaayurveda.us/wellnesscenter/doshas-what-are-they-and-how-can-they-transform-your-health/

Burtchell, J. (2023, February 3). *8 natural home remedies for knee pain.* Healthline. https://www.healthline.com/health/pain-relief/knee-pain-home-remedies

CPT, A. M. W., & CPT, C. S. (2022b, March 3). 17 Amazing Pilates exercises that work your Core—And you can do right at home. *SELF.* https://www.self.com/gallery/pilates-exercises-that-work-your-core

DePaul, K. (2021, October 11). *What does it really take to build a new habit?* Harvard Business Review. https://hbr.org/2021/02/what-does-it-really-take-to-build-a-new-habit

Fitness, O. (2023, August 25). *How many exercises should you do per workout | OPEX Fitness*. OPEX Fitness. https://www.opexfit.com/blog/how-many-exercises-should-you-do-in-a-workout

Frazier, R. S. (2023, January 7). Hit all major muscles with this 6-Move Full-Body kettlebell workout. *Health.* https://www.health.com/fitness/kettlebell-workout

Kirgios, E., Mandel, G. H., Park, Y., Milkman, K. L., Gromet, D. M., Kay, J. S., & Duckworth, A. (2020). Teaching temptation bundling to boost exercise: A field experiment. *Organizational Behavior and Human Decision Processes, 161,* 20–35. https://doi.org/10.1016/j.obhdp.2020.09.003

Nguyen US, Zhang Y, Zhu Y, Niu J, Zhang B, Felson DT. Increasing prevalence of knee pain and symptomatic knee osteoarthritis: survey and cohort data. *Ann Intern Med.* 2011;155(11):725-732.

One-minute bursts of activity during daily tasks could prolong your life. (2022, December 22). ScienceDaily. https://www.sciencedaily.com/releases/2022/12/221208114715.htm

OpenAI. (2023). ChatGPT (GTP-4) [Software]. OpenAI. https://www.openai.com

Research shows that short, intense workouts are beneficial. (n.d.). UCLA Health. https://www.uclahealth.org/news/research-shows-short-intense-workouts-are-beneficial#:~:text=Meanwhile%2C%20a%20recent

%20body%20of,more%20beneficial%20than%20extended%20ones

Tone and Tighten. (2023b, September 7). *Quick morning stretching routine for flexibility, mobility, and stiffness!* [Video]. YouTube. https://www.youtube.com/watch?v=t2jel6q1GRk

Travers, C. (2021, May 13). Is a 15-Minute workout enough to build muscle? | POPSUGAR Fitness. *POPSUGAR Fitness.* https://www.popsugar.com/fitness/is-15-minute-workout-enough-to-build-muscle-47490279

Valdez, E. (2021, April 14). *How often should you change your workout routine to maximize results?* UPPPER Gear. https://uppper.com/blogs/news/how-often-should-you-change-your-workout-routine-to-maximize-results#:~:text=Just%20remember%2C%20keep%20practicing%20indicator,trying%20to%20increase%20muscle%20mass